Sexual Harassment

SEXUAL HARASSMENT

1. Any person who practices sexual harassment in a work place, institution of learning or elsewhere on a child commits a felony and is liable, upon conviction, to imprisonment to a term of not less than three years and not exceeding fifteen years.
2. A Child who commits an offence under section (1) is liable to such community service or counseling as the court may determine in the best interest of the child.
3. In this section, sexual harassment means;

    a. A seductive sexual advance being unsolicited sexual comment, physical contact or other gesture of a sexual nature which one finds objectionable or offensive or causes discomfort in one's studies or job and interferes with academic performance or work performance or a conducive working environment or study environment;

    b. Sexual bribery in the form of soliciting or attempting to solicit sexual activity by promise of reward;

    c. Sexual threat or coercion which includes procuring or attempting to procure sexual activity by threat of violence or victimization or;

    d. Sexual imposition using forceful behavior or assault in an attempt to gain physical sexual contact.

A Child means a person below the Age of 16 years

Every Elegant Pretty Woman was Once a Girl Child

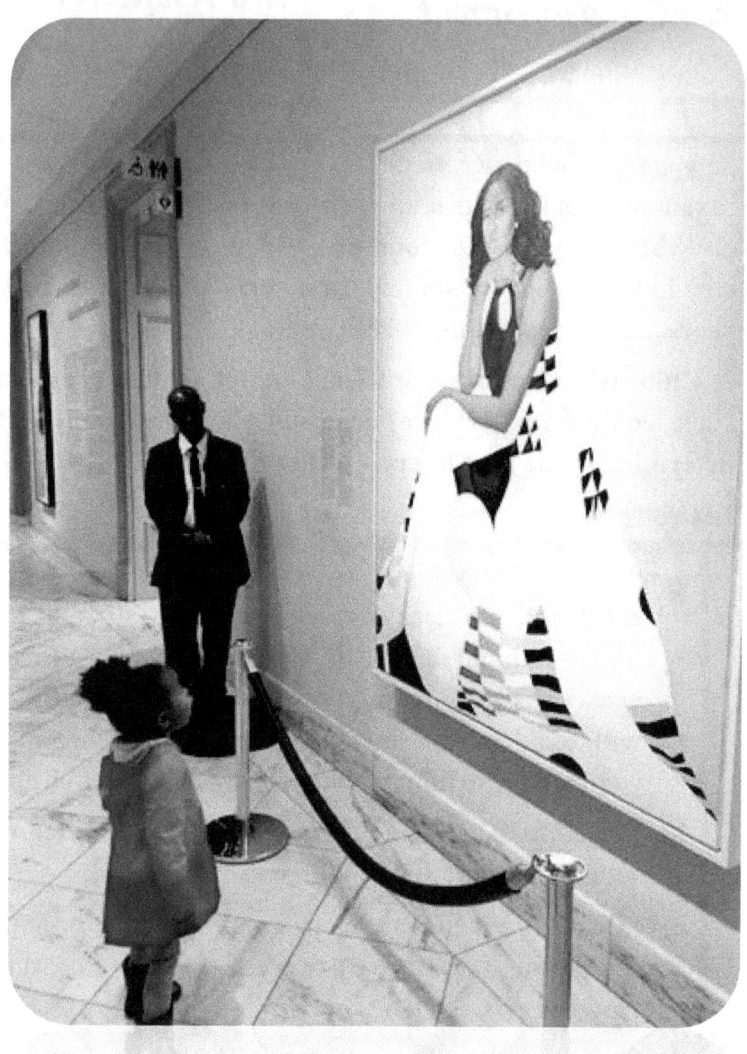

This Book is recommended for the Girl Child aged 11 to 22 as well as women of all ages

Forty percent of gynecological complaints by teen girls, young women & older women include complaints about disorders of the menstrual cycle

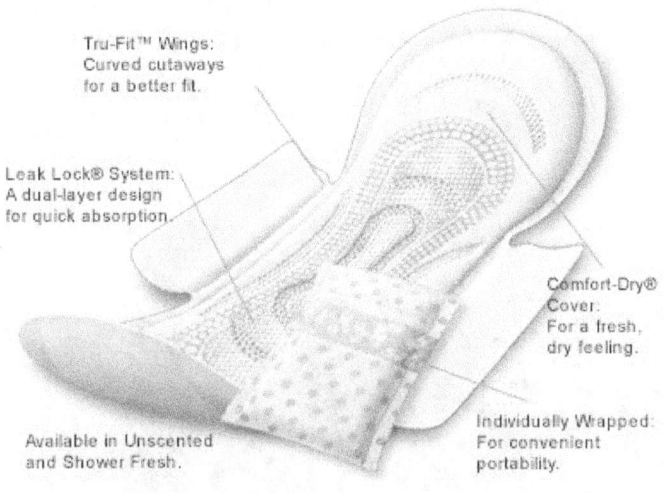

The Menstrual Cycle has Power to influence the performance of a Girl Child at School

Everyone expects her to hurriedly learn to manage herself and navigate the complex world around her. She is often judged harshly when she stumbles and Falls

Personal Tracker

Girl Child Menstrual Care Book

Girls' Health in Everyday Life

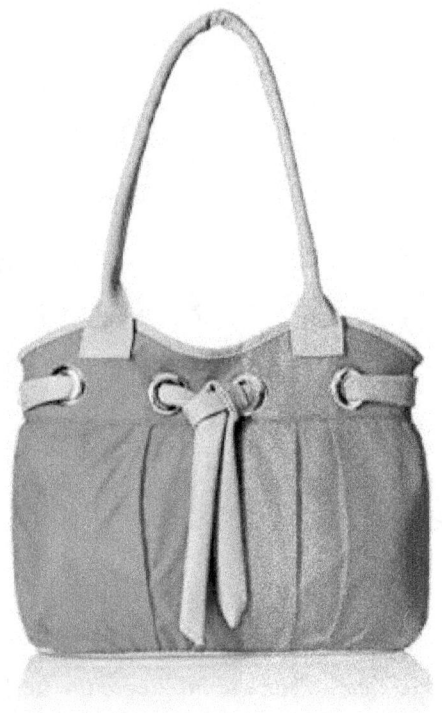

Inspired by a Girl Child

Dr K C Moonga

© Kelvin Moonga 2016

ALL RIGHTS RESERVED.

No part of this publication may be used or reproduced in any manner whatsoever without written permission except for that provided for by the publisher.

The Author and the publisher disclaim responsibility for any adverse effects resulting directly or indirectly from suggested procedures, from undetected errors, or from the reader's misunderstanding of the text.

Furthermore, the Author and publisher do not accept responsibility from emotional or other damages caused by copying or imitation of actions demonstrated in this book.

Acknowledgements

I sincerely acknowledge the distinguished contribution made by the following;

Girls at St. Mary's Secondary School in Livingstone; You raised practical questions & offered useful suggestions that shaped this book;
Mr. & Mrs. Morgan for sharing constructive thoughts and piloting this book & encouragement to roll it out to Girls in Schools, Workplaces and Homes country wide;

Ms. Kapalu for sharing her insights and an inspiring story about her amazing heroine, her niece, who rescued a Girl Child in grade eight; Seeing her classmate's uniform had been soiled, she told the boys in her class the headmaster wanted to see them at once. When the boys left the classroom, she and her friends came to the Aid of their classmate, saving her from an indelible scar of being laughed at and ridiculed by boys in class;
Ms Gillian Gideon for believing in this little book and kept the original manuscript to this petite book for seven years before it was published.

Including many I cannot list individually.

This little book is a fruition of your inspiring words.

DEDICATION

This Menstrual Care & GBV awareness Book is dedicated to

The Girl Child

It is also dedicated to

- **Teachers, Matrons, Guardians, Parents**
- **Grandmothers**
- **Women's Health in Everyday Life**
- **All the caring Men in the life of the Girl Child; Fathers, Uncles, Brothers & Grand Fathers, etc**

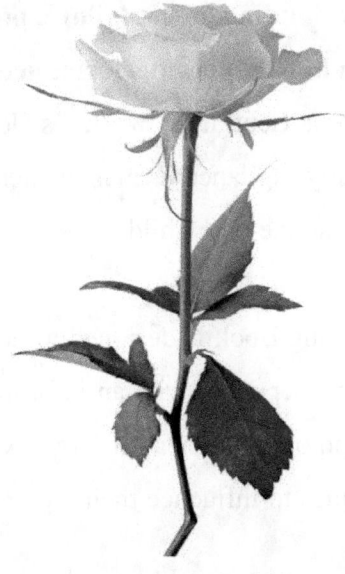

INTRODUCTION

The Menstrual Cycle is the most amazing phenomenon in the life of a woman. Its beginning, referred to as Menarche, announces monumental changes in the life of a girl child. Its end, referred to as Menopause, ushers in other monumental changes in the lives of many women. Some of these changes are so intense that they can alter a woman's personality. This can affect her social functioning beginning at home, school and work places.

The Adolescent Girl Child needs special education to understand the hormonal storm raging inside her young and naive body. Everyone expects her to hurriedly learn to manage herself and navigate the complex world around her. She is often judged harshly when she stumbles and falls.

The menstrual cycle causes her to lose blood every Month. This may cause her Anemia, a medical condition that is characterized by; poor concentration, headaches, dizziness, weakness, getting tired easily, reduced mental capacity, low immunity, poor wound healing, poor appetite, lethargy, fainting, heart failure, poor oxygen delivery to body organs, poor skin health, poor performance in school, etc.

The Menstrual Cycle is Central to Women's Health in Everyday Life; its understanding, monthly vigilance & management, is the responsibility of every Lady, Woman and the Girl Child.

This Menstrual Coloring Book is designed to help the Girl Child learn the ever changing tides in her cycle with an informed mind. It is intended to generate interest among women to re examine this powerful phenomenon that continues to influence their lives and those around them even long after it is gone.

Table of Contents

- Example — 10
1. January — 13
2. February — 17
3. March — 21
4. April — 25
5. May — 29
6. June — 33
7. July — 37
8. August — 41
9. September — 45
10. October — 49
11. November — 53
12. December — 57
13. Should I Worry about Breast Lumps — 63
14. My First Experience — 73
15. Gender Based Violence and You — 78

Example

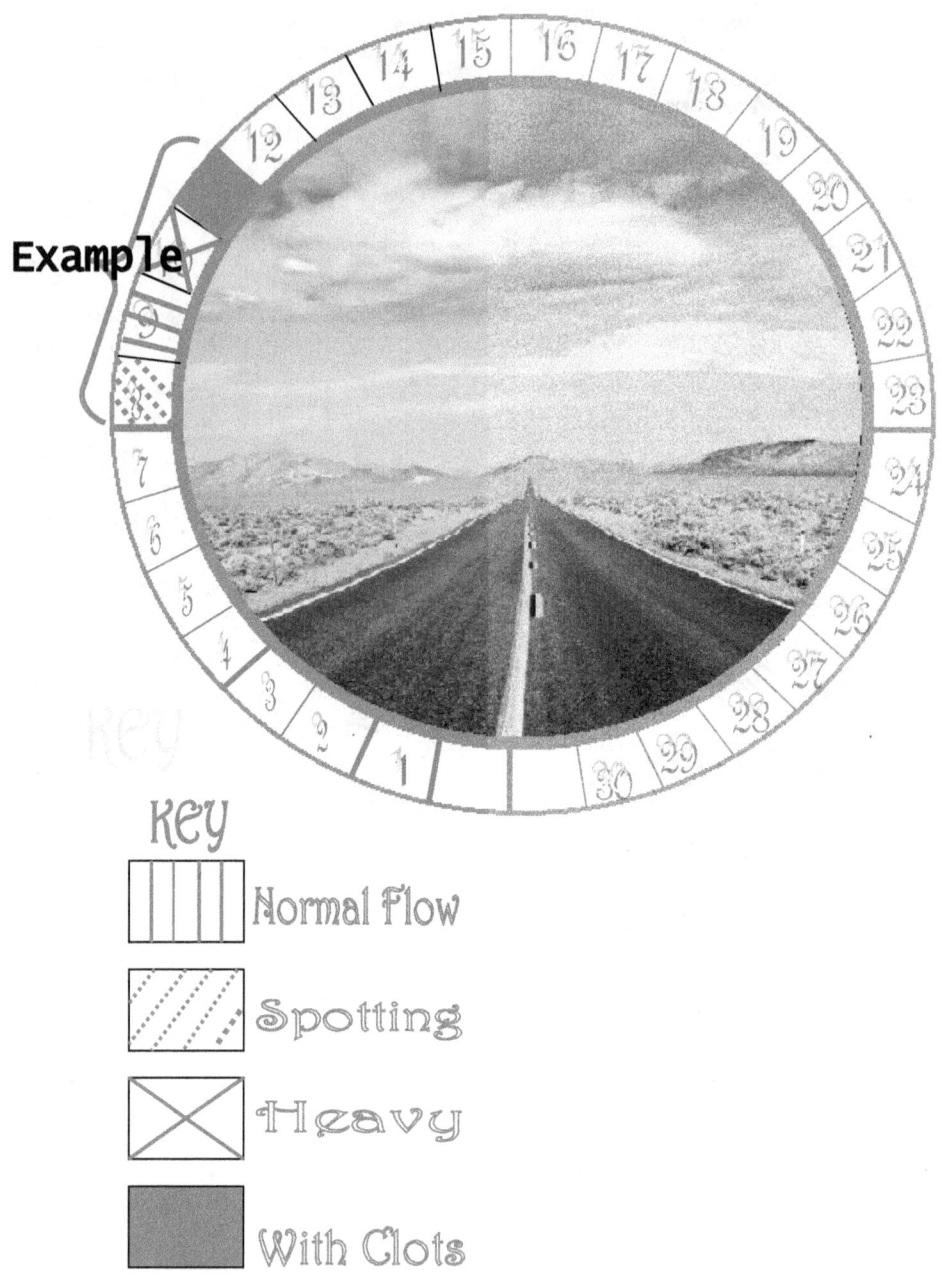

Example

Key

	Normal Flow
	Spotting
	Heavy
	With Clots

- The Average duration of normal Menses is 3 – 7 days
- The length of a normal cycle is between 21 to 35 days
- The normal Blood Loss per cycle ranges between 13 to 80 milliliters
- A Soaked standard Pad or Tampon absorbs 5 to 15 milliliters of blood

You can use this information to estimated blood loss per cycle.

Day of Menses	# of Standard Pads used	Or Number of Tampons used	Improvised Pads used
	SOAKED (x)	NOT SOAKED (y)	Nil
Day 1		2 pads	
Day 2	1 pad	3 tampons	
Day 3	3 tampons	1 pad	
Day 4	3 pads	1 pad	
Day 5		2 tampons	
Day 6			
Day 7			
TOTAL	7	9	

In the following pages, you can now follow your cycle and consult your doctor for medical advice whenever the cycle causes you concern. You can color the cycle with your favourite decor and make it stand out.

***

SHOW THIS BOOK TO YOUR HEALTH CARE PROVIDER

DURING MENSTRUAL HEALTH CONSULTATION

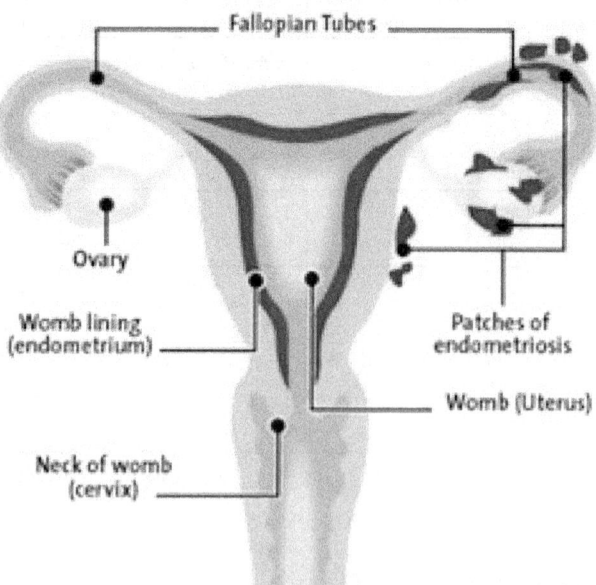

January 20......

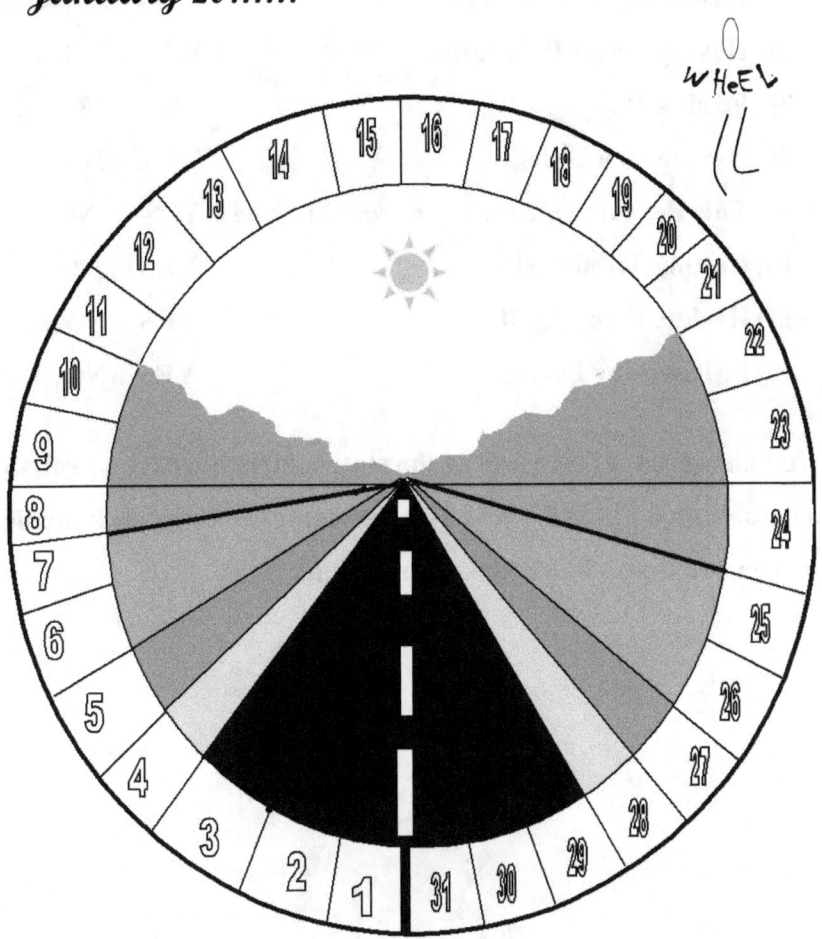

In this Cycle (Tick were appropriate)

1) Period lasted longer than seven days   YES.... NO...
2) Used more pads than is usual for me   YES..... NO...
3) Used more tampons than is usual for me YES..... NO....
4) I Bled with Clots   YES.... NO....

Personal Tracker

5) I used improvised Pads   YES... NO...
6) Having Heart Palpitations   YES... NO...
7) Feeling Dizzy   YES... NO ....
8) Having Blackouts   YES... NO...
9) This Period came too soon from last one   YES..... NO....
10) Getting Tired easily   YES... NO...
11) HB less than 10g/dl   YES...NO....
12) I Missed my Period   YES...NO...

If you answered YES to any of the statements above, you probably lost too much blood in this cycle. It is recommended you seek medical advice. You could also be at Risk of Infection.

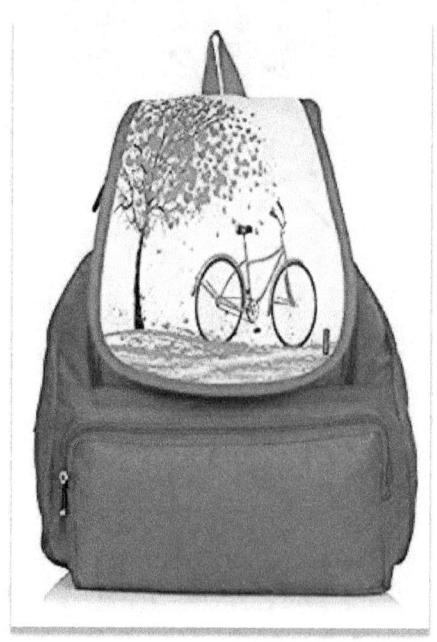

Before you go, Record the number of Pads used in this Cycle in the Table below:

Day of Menses	# of Standard Pads used	Or Number of Tampons used	# Improvised Pads used
	SOAKED (x)	NOT SOAKED (y)	
Day 1			
Day 2			
Day 3			
Day 4			
Day 5			
Day 6			
Day 7			
	Total:	Total :	

Which of the Following Complaints did you experience 7 to 10 days before your period?

1) Breast PAIN   YES/ NO
2) Vomiting   YES/NO

Personal Tracker

3) NAUSEA — YES/NO
4) HEADACHE — YES/NO
5) DEPRESSION or Feeling Low Spirited — YES/NO
6) LOSS OF APPETITE — YES/NO
7) CONSTIPATION — YES/NO
8) BACKACHE — YES/NO
9) ANGER — YES/NO
10) IRRITABLE — YES/NO
11) AGITATION — YES/NO
12) LACK OF SELF CONTROL — YES/NO
13) DIFFICULTIES WITH CONCENTRATION — YES/NO
14) TIREDNESS — YES/NO
15) INSOMNIA — YES/NO
16) WRITE OTHER COMPLAINTS YOU MAY EXPERIENCE WHICH ARE NOT LISTED ABOVE

If you answered YES to most of these statements, you probably experienced pre menstrual tension or could be suffering from pre menstrual syndrome. Consult your gyneacologist for advise.

1. COST OF SANITARY PADS/TAMPONS USED THIS MONTH: ………………..

2. BUDGET FOR PADS/TAMPONS NEXT MONTH: ……..

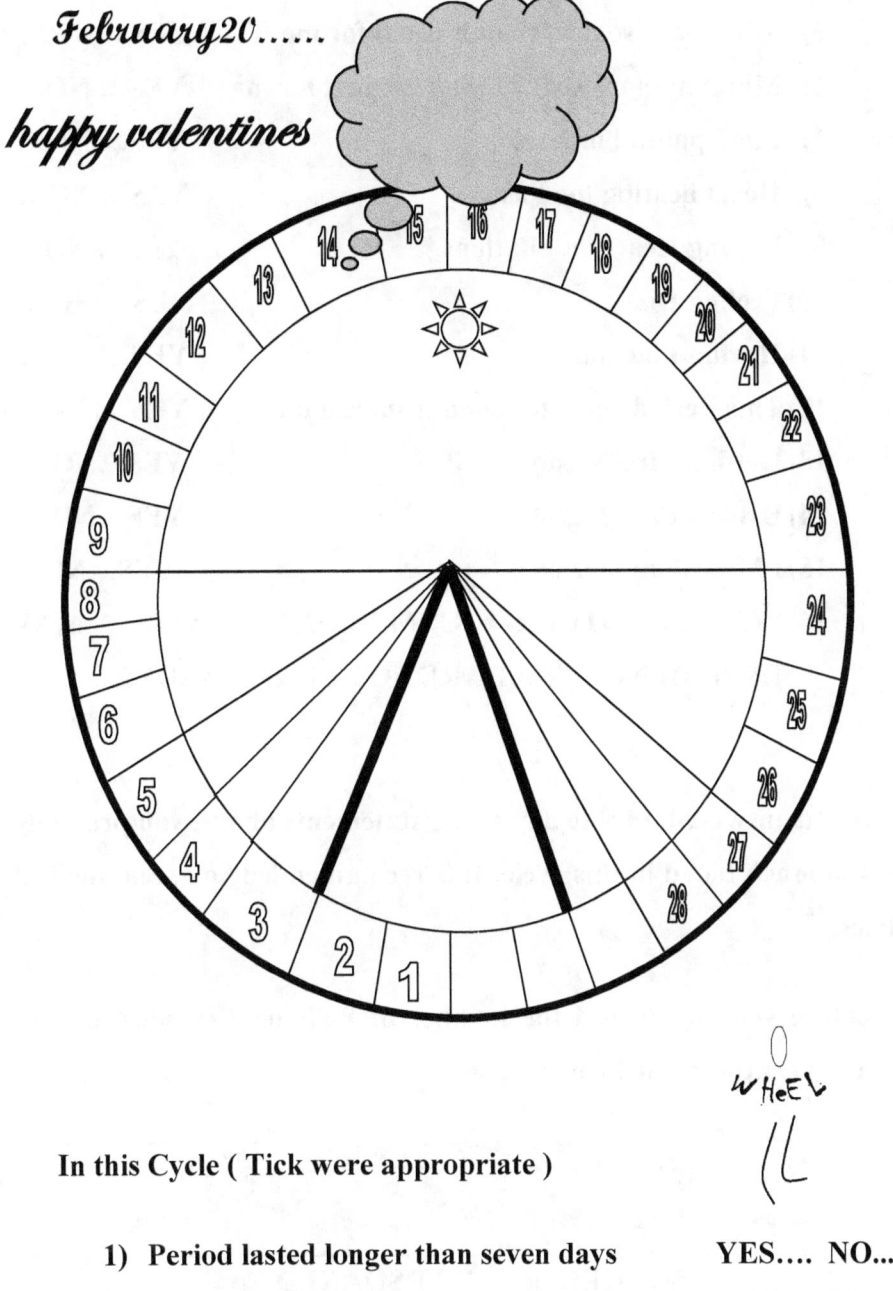

February 20......

happy valentines

WHeEL

In this Cycle (Tick were appropriate)

1) Period lasted longer than seven days   YES…. NO...
2) Used more pads than is usual for me   YES….. NO…
3) Used more tampons than is usual for me   YES….. NO….
4) I used Improvised pads   YES….. NO….

Personal Tracker

5) More pads soaked than is usual for me	YES... NO...
6) More tampons soaked than is usual for me	YES... NO...
7) I had painful menses	YES... NO...
8) Heart beating too Fast	YES... NO...
9) Having Heart Palpitations	YES... NO...
10) Feeling Dizzy	YES... NO ...
11) Having Blackouts	YES... NO...
12) This Period came too soon from last one	YES.... NO...
13) Getting Tired easily	YES...NO...
14) HB less than 10g/dl	YES...NO...
15) I Missed my Period	YES...NO...

16) WRITE OTHER COMPLAINTS YOU MAY EXPERIENCE THAT ARE NOT LISTED ABOVE

If you answered YES to any of the statements above, you probably lost too much blood in this cycle. It is recommended you seek medical advice.

Before you go, Record the number of Pads or Tampons used in this Cycle in the Table below:

Day of Menses	*# of Standard Pads used*	*Or Number of Tampons used*	# Improvised Pads used
	SOAKED (*x*)	NOT SOAKED (*y*)	
Day 1			
Day 2			

Day 3			
Day 4			
Day 5			
Day 6			
Day 7			
	Total:	Total :	

Which of the Following Complaints did you experience 7 to 10 days before your period?

    1) Breast PAIN   YES/ NO

    2) Vomiting   YES/NO

Personal Tracker

3) NAUSEA	YES/NO
4) HEADACHE	YES/NO
5) DEPRESSION or Feeling Low Spirited	YES/NO
6) LOSS OF APPETITE	YES/NO
7) CONSTIPATION	YES/NO
8) BACKACHE	YES/NO
9) ANGER	YES/NO
10) IRRITABLE	YES/NO
11) AGITATION	YES/NO
12) LACK OF SELF CONTROL	YES/NO
13) DIFFICULTIES WITH CONCENTRATION	YES/NO
14) TIREDNESS	YES/NO
15) INSOMNIA	YES/NO

If you answered YES to most of these statements, you probably experienced pre Menstrual tension or could be suffering from pre menstrual syndrome. Consult your gyneacologist for advice.

1. COST OF SANITARY PADS/TAMPONS USED THIS MONTH: ……

2. BUDGET FOR PADS/TAMPONS NEXT MONTH: ……

March 20......

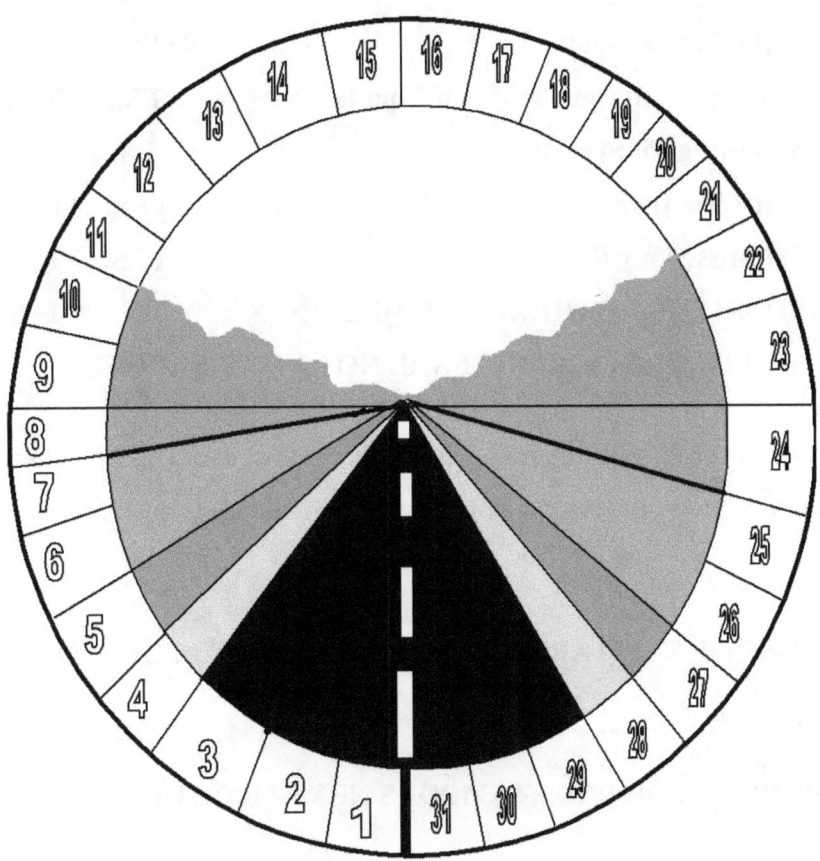

In this Cycle (Tick were appropriate)

1) Period lasted longer than seven days   YES... NO...
2) Used more pads than is usual for me   YES... NO...
3) Used more tampons than is usual for me   YES... NO...
4) I Bled with Clots   YES... NO...
5) More pads soaked than is usual for me   YES... NO...
6) More tampons soaked than is usual for me   YES... NO...
7) I used improvised Pads   YES... NO...

8) Heart beating too Fast   YES... NO...
9) Having Heart Palpitations   YES... NO...
10) Feeling Dizzy   YES... NO ...
11) Having Blackouts   YES... NO...
12) This Period came too soon from last one   YES.... NO...
13) Getting Tired easily   YES...NO...
14) HB less than 10g/dl   YES...NO...
15) I Missed my Period   YES...NO...
16) WRITE OTHER COMPLAINTS YOU MAY EXPERIENCE WHICH ARE NOT LISTED ABOVE

If you answered YES to any of the statements above, you probably lost too much blood in this cycle. It is recommended you seek medical advice.

1. COST OF SANITARY PADS/TAMPONS USED THIS MONTH: ……………..
2. BUDGET FOR PADS/TAMPONS NEXT MONTH: ……..

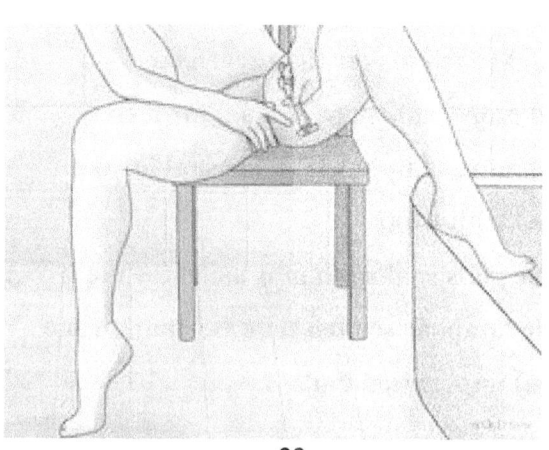

Before you go, Record the number of Pads used in this Cycle in the Table below:

Day of Menses	# of Standard Pads used	Or Number of Tampons used	# Improvised Pads used
	SOAKED (x)	NOT SOAKED (y)	
Day 1			
Day 2			
Day 3			
Day 4			
Day 5			
Day 6			
Day 7			
	Total:	Total :	

Which of the Following Complaints did you experience 7 to 10 days before your period?

1) Breast PAIN — YES/ NO
2) Vomiting — YES/NO
3) NAUSEA — YES/NO
4) HEADACHE — YES/NO

Personal Tracker

5) DEPRESSION or Feeling Low Spirited	YES/NO
6) LOSS OF APPETITE	YES/NO
7) CONSTIPATION	YES/NO
8) BACKACHE	YES/NO
9) ANGER	YES/NO
10) IRRITABLE	YES/NO
11) AGITATION	YES/NO
12) LACK OF SELF CONTROL	YES/NO
13) DIFFICULTIES WITH CONCENTRATION	YES/NO
14) TIREDNESS	YES/NO
15) INSOMNIA	YES/NO
16) I FEEL LUMPS IN MY BREASTS	YES/NO

17) WRITE OTHER COMPLAINTS YOU MAY EXPERIENCE WHICH ARE NOT LISTED ABOVE

If you answered YES to most of these statements, you probably experienced pre Menstrual tension or could be suffering from pre menstrual syndrome. Consult your gyneacologist for advice. See a Surgeon or Nurse for advice on Lumps in Your Breast.

April 20......

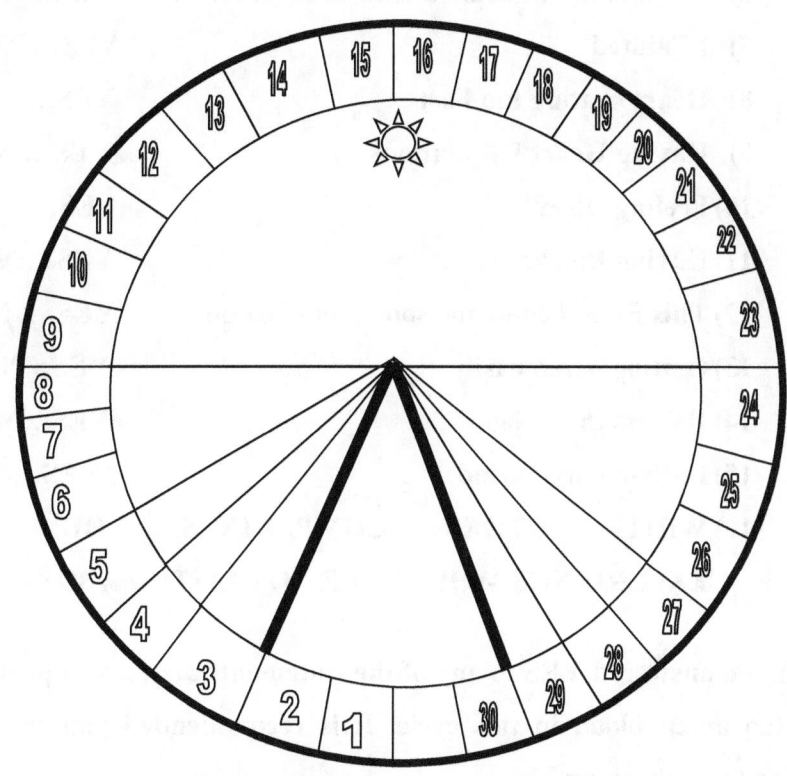

In this Cycle (Tick were appropriate)

1) Period lasted longer than seven days   YES... NO...
2) Used more pads than is usual for me   YES... NO...
3) Used more tampons than is usual for me YES... NO...
4) I Bled with Clots   YES... NO...

Personal Tracker

5) More pads soaked than is usual for me   YES... NO...
6) More tampons soaked than is usual for me   YES... NO...
7) I Fainted   YES... NO...
8) Heart beating too Fast   YES... NO...
9) Having Heart Palpitations   YES... NO...
10) Feeling Dizzy   YES... NO...
11) Having Blackouts   YES... NO...
12) This Period came too soon from last one   YES.... NO...
13) Getting Tired easily   YES...NO...
14) HB less than 10g/dl   YES...NO...
15) I Missed my Period   YES...NO...
16) WRITE OTHER COMPLAINTS YOU MAY EXPERIENCE WHICH ARE NOT LISTED ABOVE

If you answered YES to any of the statements above, you probably lost too much blood in this cycle. It is recommended you see your Doctor for a check up.

Before you go, Record the number of Pads or Tampons used in this Cycle in the Table below:

Day of Menses	# of Standard Pads used	Or Number of Tampons used	# Improvised Pads used
	SOAKED (x)	NOT SOAKED (y)	
Day 1			

Day 2			
Day 3			
Day 4			
Day 5			
Day 6			
Day 7			
	Total:	Total :	

Which of the Following Complaints did you experience 7 to 10 days before your period?

1) Breast PAIN   YES/ NO
2) Vomiting   YES/NO

Personal Tracker

3) NAUSEA	YES/NO
4) HEADACHE	YES/NO
5) DEPRESSION or Feeling Low	YES/NO
6) LOSS OF APPETITE	YES/NO
7) CONSTIPATION	YES/NO
8) BACKACHE	YES/NO
9) ANGER	YES/NO
10) IRRITABLE	YES/NO
11) AGITATION	YES/NO
12) LACK OF SELF CONTROL	YES/NO
13) DIFFICULTIES WITH CONCENTRATION	YES/NO
14) TIREDNESS	YES/NO
15) INSOMNIA	YES/NO
16) I Feel Lumps in my Breasts	YES/NO

17) WRITE OTHER COMPLAINTS YOU MAY EXPERIENCE WHICH ARE NOT LISTED ABOVE

If you answered YES to most of these statements, you probably experienced pre Menstrual tension or could be suffering from pre menstrual syndrome. Consult your gyneacologist for advice. See a Surgeon or Nurse for advice on Lumps in Your Breast.

May 20......   WHeEL

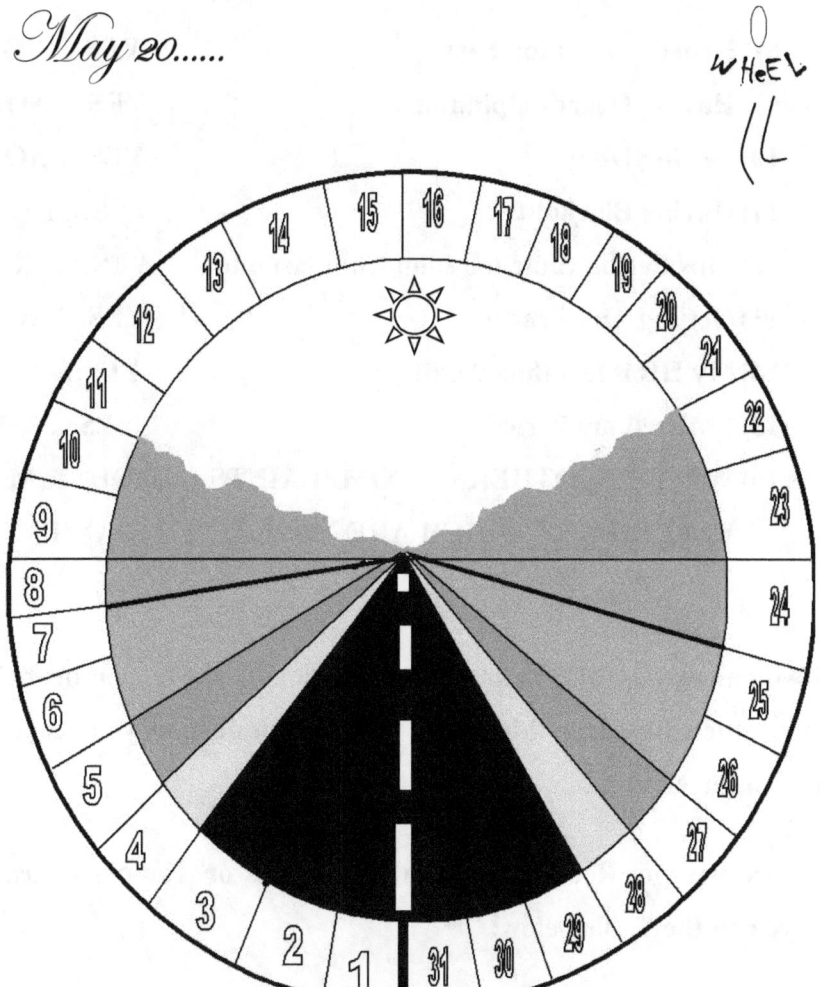

In this Cycle (Tick were appropriate)

1) Period lasted longer than seven days   YES... NO...
2) Used more pads than is usual for me   YES... NO...
3) Used more tampons than is usual for me   YES... NO...
4) I Bled with Clots   YES... NO...
5) More pads soaked than is usual for me   YES... NO...
6) More tampons soaked than is usual for me   YES... NO...
7) I lost consciousness   YES... NO...

8) Heart beating too Fast — YES… NO…
9) Having Heart Palpitations — YES… NO…
10) Feeling Dizzy — YES… NO …
11) Having Blackouts — YES… NO…
12) This Period came too soon from last one — YES…. NO…
13) Getting Tired easily — YES… NO…
14) My HB is less than 9 g/dl — YES… NO…
15) I Missed my Period — YES… NO…
16) WRITE OTHER COMPLAINTS YOU MAY EXPERIENCE WHICH ARE NOT LISTED ABOVE

If you answered YES to any of the statements above, you probably lost too much blood in this cycle. It is recommended you see your doctor for check ups.

Before you go, Record the number of Pads or Tampons used in this Cycle in the Table below:

Day of Menses	# of Standard Pads used	Or Number of Tampons used	# Improvised Pads used
	SOAKED (x)	NOT SOAKED (y)	
Day 1			
Day 2			
Day 3			
Day 4			

Day 5			
Day 6			
Day 7			
	Total:	Total :	

Which of the Following Complaints did you experience 7 to 10 days before your period?

1) Breast PAIN — YES/ NO
2) Vomiting — YES/NO
3) NAUSEA — YES/NO
4) HEADACHE — YES/NO
5) DEPRESSION or Feeling Low — YES/NO
6) LOSS OF APPETITE — YES/NO
7) CONSTIPATION — YES/NO
8) BACKACHE — YES/NO
9) ANGER — YES/NO
10) IRRITABLE — YES/NO
11) AGITATION — YES/NO
12) LACK OF SELF CONTROL — YES/NO
13) DIFFICULTIES WITH CONCENTRATION — YES/NO
14) TIREDNESS — YES/NO

15) INSOMNIA   YES/NO

16) I FEEL LUMPS IN MY BREASTS   YES/NO

17) WRITE OTHER COMPLAINTS YOU MAY EXPERIENCE WHICH ARE NOT LISTED ABOVE

If you answered YES to most of these statements, you probably experienced pre Menstrual tension or could be suffering from pre menstrual syndrome. Consult your gyneacologist for advice. See a Surgeon or Nurse for advice on Lumps in Your Breast.

WHeEL - Women's Health in Everyday Life

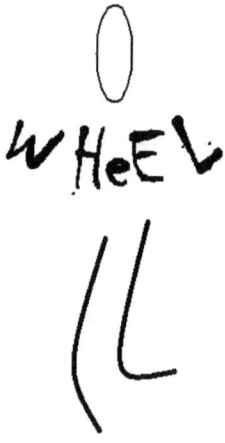

1. COST OF SANITARY PADS/TAMPONS USED THIS MONTH: ………………..

2. MY BUDGET FOR PADS/TAMPONS NEXT MONTH: …

June 20......

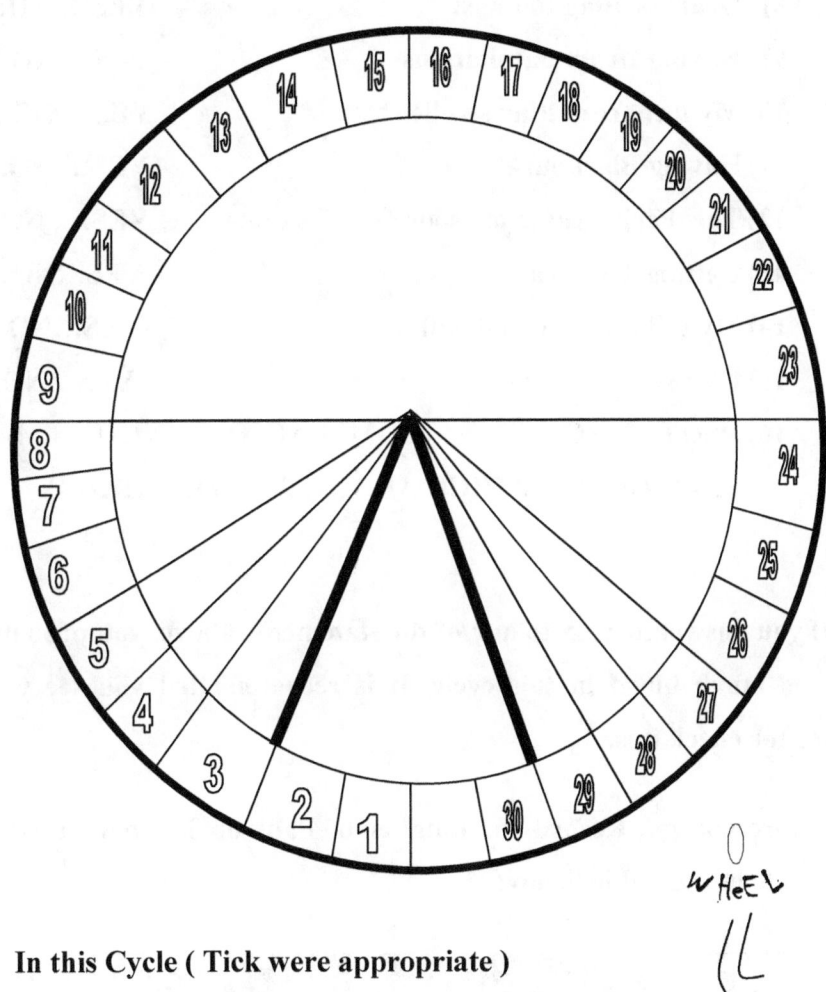

In this Cycle (Tick were appropriate)

1) Period lasted longer than seven days   YES... NO...
2) Used more pads than is usual for me   YES... NO...
3) Used more tampons than is usual for me   YES... NO...

Personal Tracker

4) I Fainted — YES... NO...
5) More pads soaked than is usual for me — YES... NO...
6) More tampons soaked than is usual for me — YES... NO...
7) Bleeding with Clots — YES... NO...
8) Heart beating too Fast — YES... NO...
9) Having Heart Palpitations — YES... NO...
10) My feet are getting swollen — YES... NO ...
11) Having Blackouts — YES... NO...
12) This Period came too soon from last one — YES.... NO...
13) Getting Tired easily — YES...NO...
14) My HB is less than 8 g/dl — YES...NO...
15) I Missed my Period — YES...NO...
16) WRITE OTHER COMPLAINTS YOU MAY EXPERIENCE WHICH ARE NOT LISTED ABOVE

If you answered YES to any of the statements above, you probably lost too much blood in this cycle. It is recommended you see your doctor for check ups.

Before you go, Record the number of Pads or Tampons used in this Cycle in the Table below:

Day of Menses	# of Standard Pads used	Or Number of Tampons used	# Improvised Pads used
	SOAKED (x)	NOT SOAKED (y)	
Day 1			

Day 2			
Day 3			
Day 4			
Day 5			
Day 6			
Day 7			

Which of the Following Complaints did you experience 7 to 10 days before your menses?

1) Breast PAIN   YES/ NO
2) Vomiting   YES/NO
3) NAUSEA   YES/NO
4) HEADACHE   YES/NO
5) DEPRESSION or Feeling Low   YES/NO
6) LOSS OF APPETITE   YES/NO
7) CONSTIPATION   YES/NO
8) BACKACHE   YES/NO
9) ANGER   YES/NO
10) IRRITABLE   YES/NO
11) AGITATION   YES/NO
12) LACK OF SELF CONTROL   YES/NO

13) DIFFICULTIES WITH CONCENTRATION   YES/NO
14) TIREDNESS   YES/NO
15) INSOMNIA   YES/NO
16) I FEEL LUMPS IN MY BREASTS   YES/NO
17) WRITE OTHER COMPLAINTS YOU MAY EXPERIENCE WHICH ARE NOT LISTED ABOVE

If you answered YES to most of these statements, you probably experienced pre Menstrual tension or could be suffering from pre menstrual syndrome. Consult your gyneacologist for advice. See a Surgeon or Nurse for advice on Lumps in Your Breast.

SHOW THIS BOOK TO YOUR HEALTH CARE PROVIDER DURING MENSTRUAL HEALTH CONSULTATION

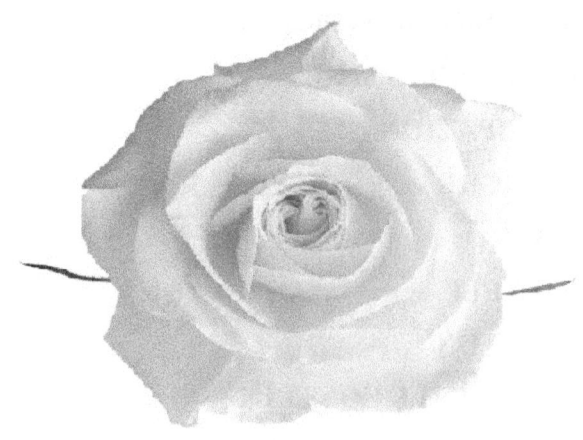

July 20......

0
1
2
3
4
5
6
7
8
9
10
11
12
13
14
15
16
17
18
19
20
21
22
23
24
25
26
27
28
29
30
31

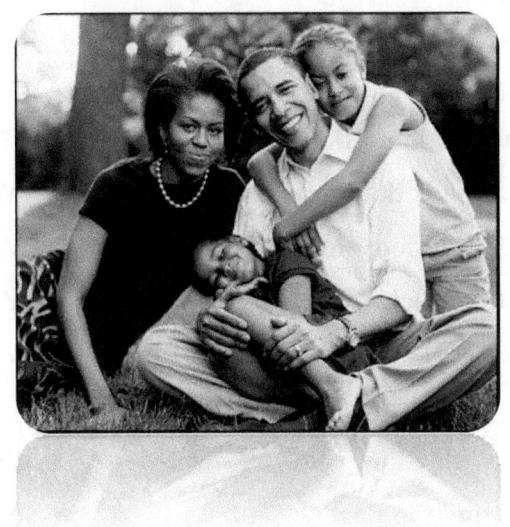

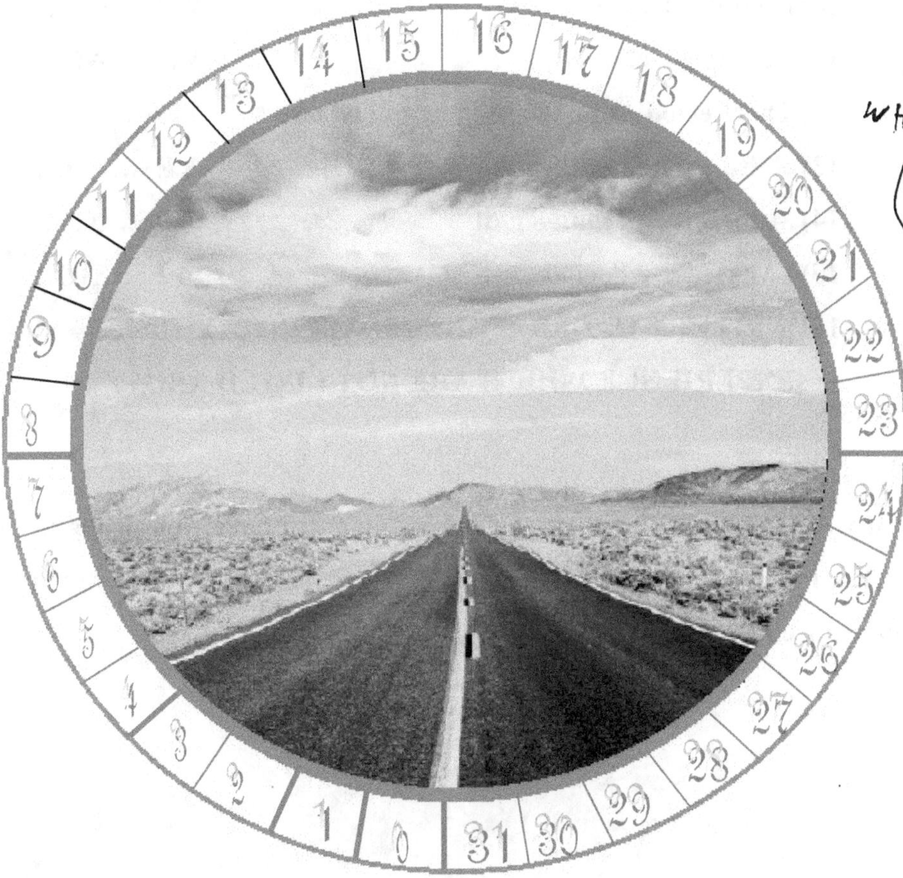

Personal Tracker

In this Cycle (Tick were appropriate)

1) Period lasted longer than seven days   YES... NO...
2) Used more pads than is usual for me   YES... NO...
3) Used more tampons than is usual for me   YES... NO...
4) I missed the Mock Exams   YES... NO...
5) More pads soaked than is usual for me   YES... NO...
6) More tampons soaked than is usual for me   YES... NO...
7) Bleeding with Clots   YES... NO...
8) Heart beating too Fast   YES... NO...
9) Having Heart Palpitations   YES... NO...
10) Feeling Dizzy   YES... NO ...
11) Having Blackouts   YES... NO...
12) This Period came too soon from last one   YES.... NO...
13) Getting Tired easily   YES...NO...
14) My HB is less than 8 g/dl   YES...NO...
15) I Missed my Period   YES...NO...
16) WRITE OTHER COMPLAINTS YOU MAY EXPERIENCE WHICH ARE NOT LISTED ABOVE

If you answered YES to any of the statements above, you probably lost too much blood in this cycle. It is recommended you see your doctor for check ups.

Before you go, Record the number of Pads or Tampons used in this Cycle in the Table below:

Day of Menses	# of Standard Pads used	Or Number of Tampons used	# Improvised Pads used
	SOAKED (x)	NOT SOAKED (y)	
Day 1			
Day 2			
Day 3			
Day 4			
Day 5			
Day 6			
Day 7			
	Total:	Total :	

Which of the Following Complaints did you experience 7 to 10 days before your menses?

1) Breast PAIN   YES/ NO
2) Vomiting   YES/NO
3) NAUSEA   YES/NO
4) HEADACHE   YES/NO

Personal Tracker

5) DEPRESSION or Feeling Low — YES/NO
6) LOSS OF APPETITE — YES/NO
7) CONSTIPATION — YES/NO
8) BACKACHE — YES/NO
9) ANGER — YES/NO
10) IRRITABLE — YES/NO
11) AGITATION — YES/NO
12) LACK OF SELF CONTROL — YES/NO
13) DIFFICULTIES WITH CONCENTRATION — YES/NO
14) TIREDNESS — YES/NO
15) INSOMNIA — YES/NO
16) I FEEL LUMPS IN MY BREASTS — YES/NO
17) WRITE OTHER COMPLAINTS YOU MAY EXPERIENCE WHICH ARE NOT LISTED ABOVE

If you answered YES to most of these statements, you probably experienced pre Menstrual tension or could be suffering from Pre Menstrual Syndrome (PMS). Consult your gyneacologist for advice. See a Surgeon or Nurse for advice on Lumps in Your Breast.

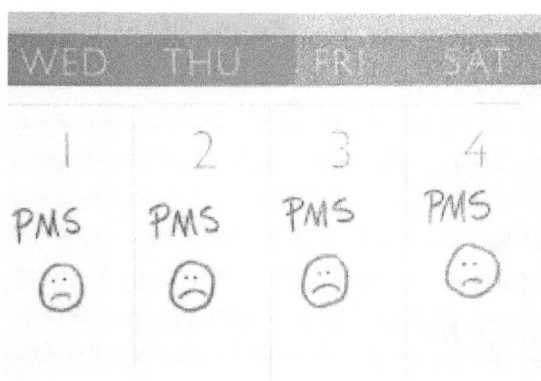

August 20......

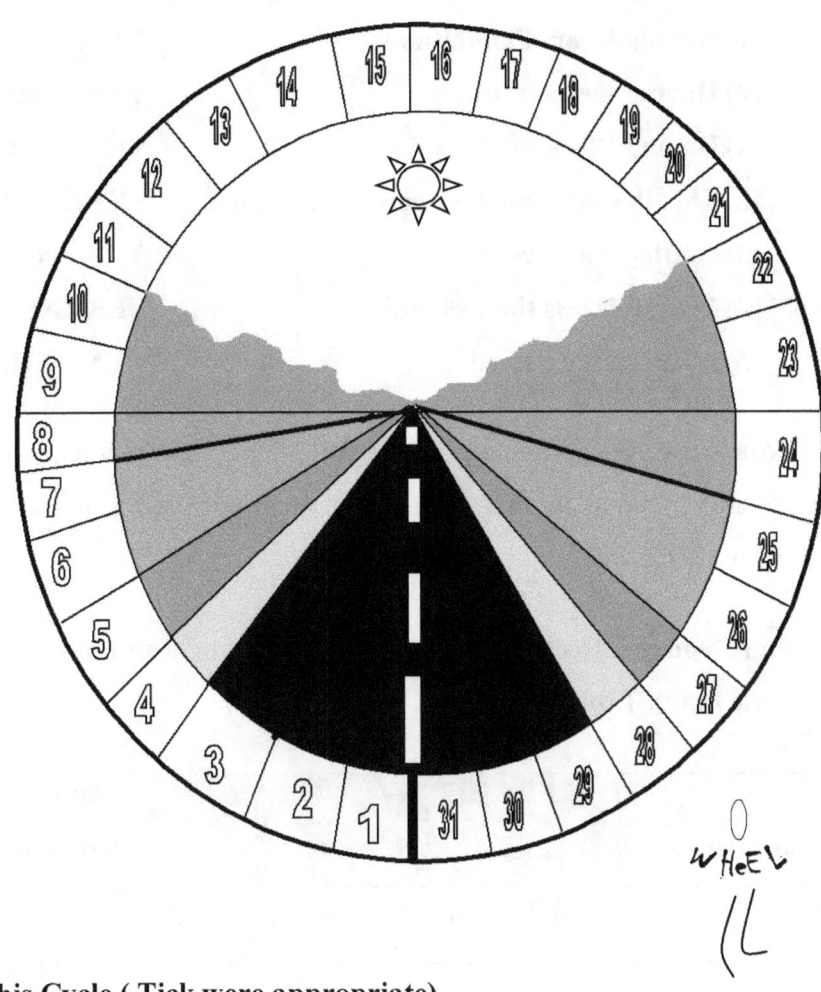

In this Cycle (Tick were appropriate)

1) Period lasted longer than seven days   YES... NO...
2) Used more pads than is usual for me   YES... NO...
3) Used more tampons than is usual for me   YES... NO...
4) I was admitted to hospital   YES... NO...
5) More pads soaked than is usual for me   YES... NO...

Personal Tracker

6) More tampons soaked than is usual for me	YES... NO...
7) Bleeding with Clots	YES... NO...
8) Having severe abdominal & back pain	YES... NO...
9) Having Heart Palpitations	YES... NO...
10) Having nose bleeds	YES... NO ...
11) Having Blackouts	YES... NO...
12) This Period came too soon from last one	YES.... NO...
13) Getting Tired easily	YES...NO...
14) My HB is less than 10 g/dl	YES...NO...
15) I Missed my Period	YES...NO...

If you answered YES to any of the statements above, you probably lost too much blood in this cycle. It is recommended you see your doctor for check ups.

Before you go, Record the number of Pads or Tampons used in this Cycle in the Table below:

Day of Menses	*# of Standard Pads used*	*Or Number of Tampons used*	# Improvised Pads used
	SOAKED (*x*)	NOT SOAKED (*y*)	
Day 1			
Day 2			
Day 3			
Day 4			
Day 5			

Day 6			
Day 7			
	Total:	Total :	

Which of the Following Complaints did you experience 7 to 10 days before your menses?

1) Breast PAIN — YES/ NO
2) Vomiting — YES/NO
3) NAUSEA — YES/NO
4) HEADACHE — YES/NO
5) DEPRESSION or Feeling Low Spirited — YES/NO
6) LOSS OF APPETITE — YES/NO
7) CONSTIPATION — YES/NO
8) BACKACHE — YES/NO
9) ANGER — YES/NO
10) IRRITABLE — YES/NO
11) AGITATION — YES/NO
12) LACK OF SELF CONTROL — YES/NO
13) DIFFICULTIES WITH CONCENTRATION — YES/NO
14) TIREDNESS — YES/NO
15) INSOMNIA — YES/NO
16) LUMPS IN MY BREASTS — YES/NO

17) WRITE OTHER COMPLAINTS YOU MAY EXPERIENCE WHICH ARE NOT LISTED ABOVE

If you answered YES to most of these statements, you probably experienced pre Menstrual tension or could be suffering from pre menstrual syndrome. Consult your gyneacologist for advice. See a SURGEON or Nurse for advice on Lumps in Your Breast.

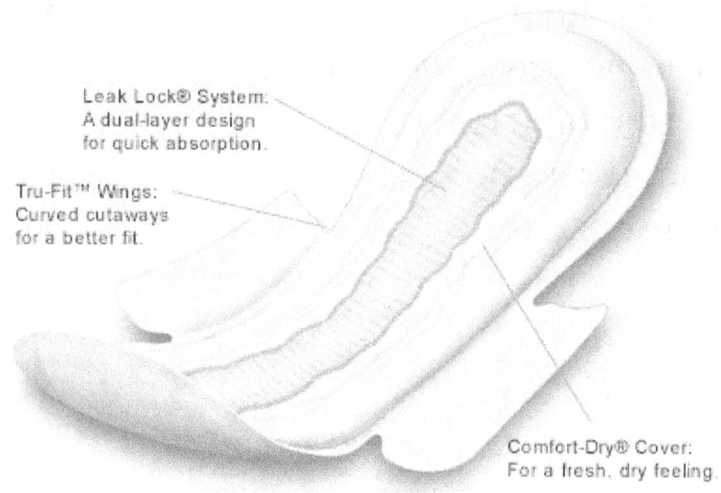

September 20......

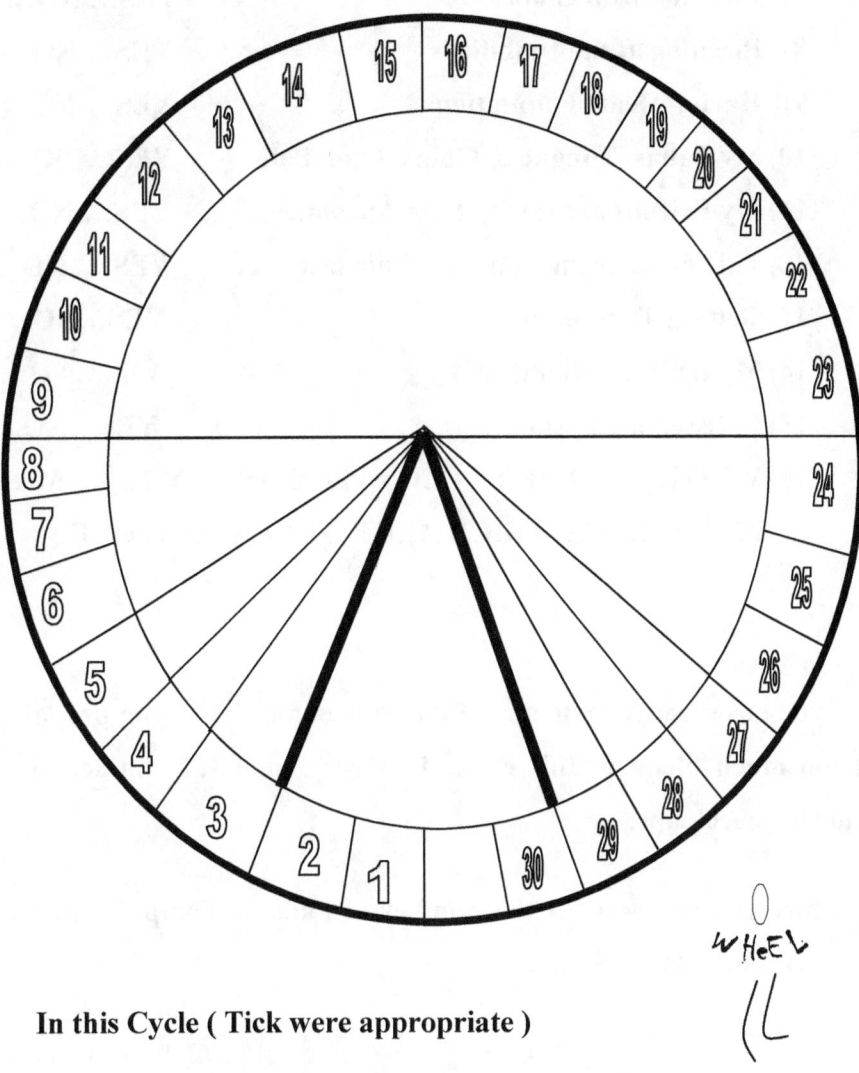

In this Cycle (Tick were appropriate)

    1) Period lasted longer than seven days   YES... NO...

    2) Used more pads than is usual for me   YES... NO...

    3) Used more tampons than is usual for me   YES... NO...

    4) I Nearly Died   YES... NO...

    5) More pads soaked than is usual for me   YES... NO...

Personal Tracker

6) More tampons soaked than is usual for me   YES... NO...
7) Bleeding with Clots   YES... NO...
8) Bleeding at the Umbilicus   YES... NO...
9) Having Heart Palpitations   YES... NO...
10) My Palms, Tongue & Gums Look Pale   YES... NO ...
11) My Friends are saying I am Aneamic   YES... NO...
12) This Period came too soon from last one   YES.... NO...
13) Getting Tired easily   YES...NO...
14) My HB is less than 7 g/dl   YES...NO...
15) I Missed my Period   YES...NO...
16) WRITE OTHER COMPLAINTS YOU MAY EXPERIENCE WHICH ARE NOT LISTED ABOVE

If you answered YES to any of the statements above, you probably lost too much blood in this cycle. It is recommended you see your doctor for check ups.

Before you go, Record the number of Pads or Tampons used in this Cycle in the table below:

Day of Menses	# of Standard Pads used	Or Number of Tampons used	# Improvised Pads used
	SOAKED (x)	NOT SOAKED (y)	
Day 1			
Day 2			

Day 3			
Day 4			
Day 5			
Day 6			
Day 7			
	Total:	Total :	

Which of the Following Complaints did you experience 7 to 10 days before your menses?

1) Breast PAIN — YES/ NO
2) Vomiting — YES/NO
3) NAUSEA — YES/NO
4) HEADACHE — YES/NO
5) DEPRESSION or Feeling Low Spirited — YES/NO
6) LOSS OF APPETITE — YES/NO
7) CONSTIPATION — YES/NO
8) BACKACHE — YES/NO
9) ANGER — YES/NO
10) IRRITABLE — YES/NO
11) AGITATION — YES/NO

12) LACK OF SELF CONTROL YES/NO
13) DIFFICULTIES WITH CONCENTRATION YES/NO
14) TIREDNESS YES/NO
15) INSOMNIA YES/NO
16) I FEEL LUMPS IN MY BREASTS YES/NO
17) WRITE OTHER COMPLAINTS YOU MAY EXPERIENCE WHICH ARE NOT LISTED ABOVE

If you answered YES to most of these statements, you probably experienced pre Menstrual tension or could be suffering from pre menstrual syndrome. Consult your gyneacologist for advice. See a Surgeon or Nurse for advice on Lumps in Your Breast.

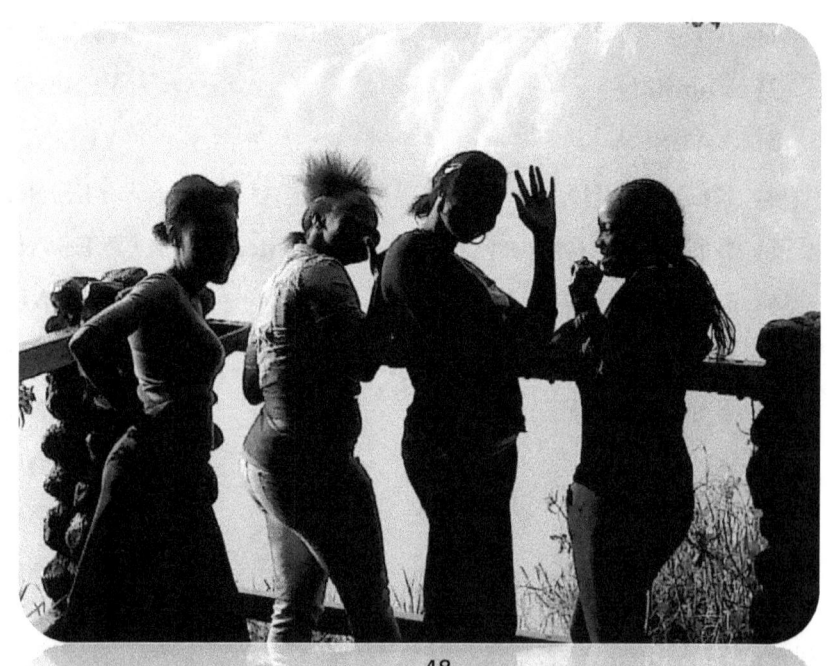

October 20......

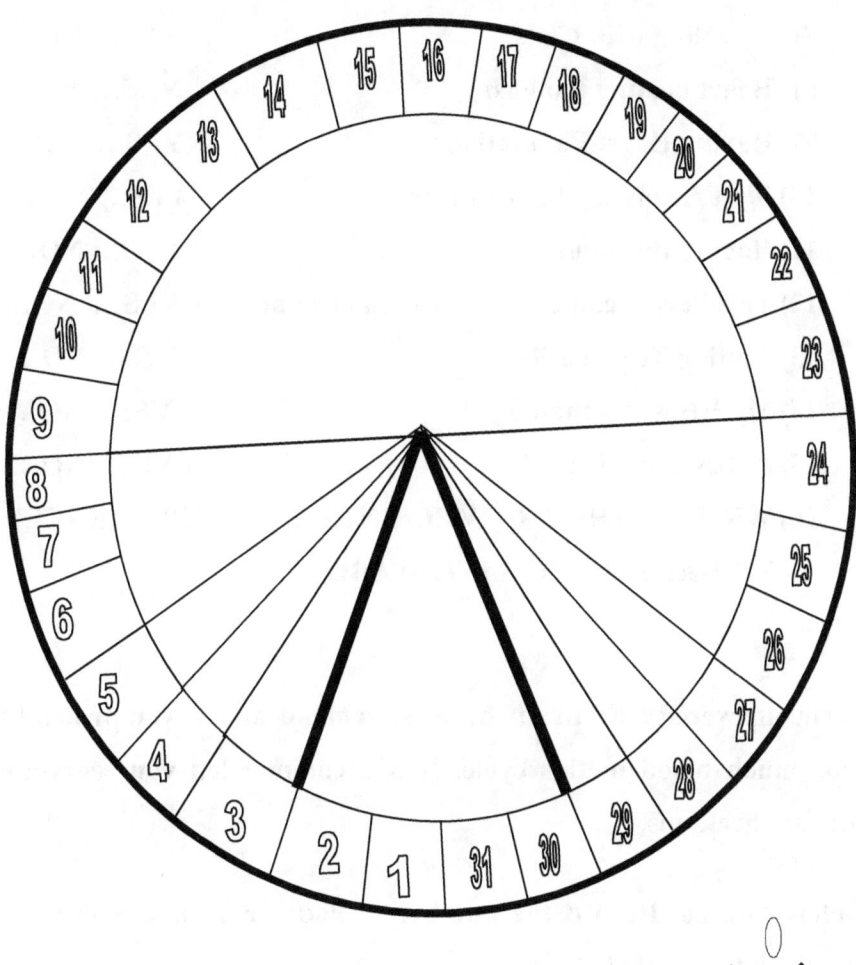

In this Cycle (Tick were appropriate)

1) Period lasted longer than seven days   YES... NO...
2) Used more pads than is usual for me   YES... NO...
3) Used more tampons than is usual for me   YES... NO...
4) I Missed School   YES... NO...

Personal Tracker

5) More pads soaked than is usual for me   YES… NO…
6) More tampons soaked than is usual for me   YES… NO…
7) Bleeding with Clots   YES… NO…
8) Heart beating too Fast   YES… NO…
9) Having Heart Palpitations   YES… NO…
10) My Friends say I am Aneamic   YES… NO …
11) Having Blackouts   YES… NO…
12) This Period came too soon from last one   YES…. NO…
13) Getting Tired easily   YES…NO…
14) My HB is less than 8 g/dl   YES…NO…
15) I Missed my Period   YES…NO…
16) WRITE OTHER COMPLAINTS YOU EXPERIENCED WHICH ARE NOT LISTED ABOVE

If you answered YES to any of the statements above, you probably lost too much blood in this cycle. It is recommended you see your doctor for check ups.

Before you go, Record the number of Pads or Tampons used in this Cycle in the Table below:

Day of Menses	# of Standard *Pads used*	Or Number of *Tampons used*	# Improvised Pads used
	SOAKED (x)	NOT SOAKED (y)	
Day 1			
Day 2			

Day 3			
Day 4			
Day 5			
Day 6			
Day 7			
	Total:	Total :	

Which of the Following Complaints did you experience 7 to 10 days before your menses?

1) Breast PAIN — YES/ NO
2) Vomiting — YES/NO
3) NAUSEA — YES/NO
4) HEADACHE — YES/NO
5) DEPRESSION or Feeling Low — YES/NO
6) LOSS OF APPETITE — YES/NO
7) CONSTIPATION — YES/NO
8) BACKACHE — YES/NO
9) ANGER — YES/NO
10) IRRITABLE — YES/NO
11) AGITATION — YES/NO
12) LACK OF SELF CONTROL — YES/NO
13) DIFFICULTIES WITH CONCENTRATION — YES/NO

14) TIREDNESS   YES/NO

15) INSOMNIA   YES/NO

16) I FEEL LUMPS IN MY BREASTS   YES/NO

17) WRITE OTHER COMPLAINTS YOU MAY EXPERIENCE WHICH ARE NOT LISTED ABOVE

If you answered YES to most of these statements, you probably experienced pre Menstrual tension or could be suffering from pre menstrual syndrome. Consult your gyneacologist for advice. See a Surgeon or Nurse for advice on Lumps in Your Breast.

1. COST OF SANITARY PADS/TAMPONS USED THIS MONTH: ………………..

2. MY BUDGET FOR PADS/TAMPONS NEXT MONTH: …

WARNING

USE OF NON STERILE IMPROVISED PADS IS UNHYGIENIC AND DANGEROUS. A Girl Child or Young Woman should only Use Recommended Sterile Sanitary Pads or Tampons. A woman is at greatest risk of Ascending Pelvic infection during her Menses. This can lead to Pelvic Inflammatory Disease (PID) and may complicate into a Pelvic Abscess, chronic pelvic pain syndrome, Ectopic Pregnancies, Infertility (Infertility is failure to conceive after a year of regular unprotected coitus usually referring to married couples)

November 20......

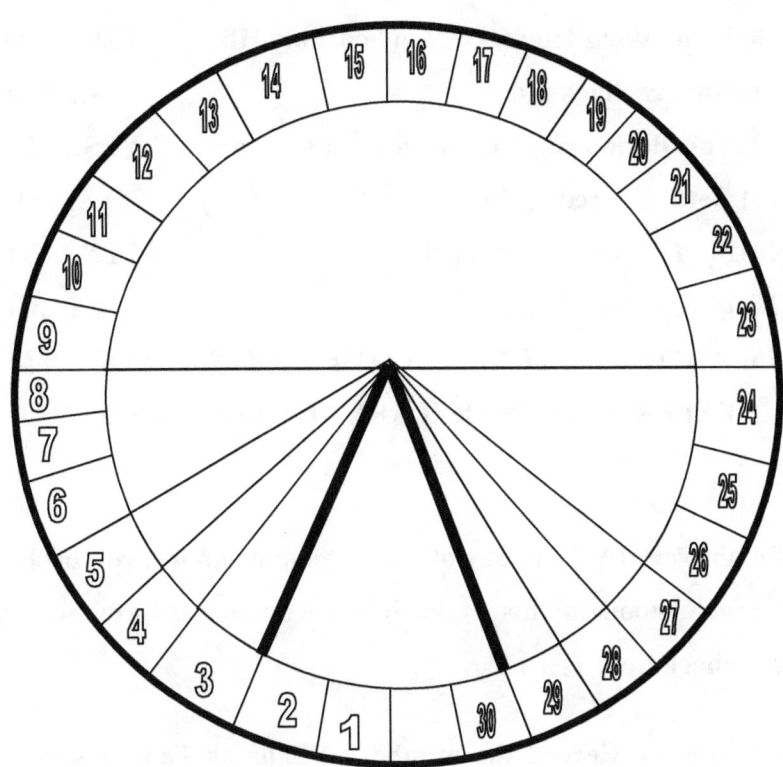

In this Cycle (Tick were appropriate)

1) Period lasted longer than seven days   YES... NO...
2) Used more pads than is usual for me   YES... NO...
3) Used more tampons than is usual for me   YES... NO...
4) I missed my Exams   YES... NO...

Personal Tracker

5) More pads soaked than is usual for me   YES… NO…
6) More tampons soaked than is usual for me   YES… NO…
7) Bleeding with Clots   YES… NO…
8) Heart beating too Fast   YES… NO…
9) Having Heart Palpitations   YES… NO…
10) I am taking Iron tablets to boost my Hb   YES… NO …
11) Having Blackouts   YES… NO…
12) This Period came too soon from last one   YES…. NO…
13) Getting Tired easily   YES…NO…
14) My HB is less than 8 g/dl   YES…NO…
15) I Missed my Period   YES…NO…
16) WRITE OTHER COMPLAINTS YOU MAY EXPERIENCE WHICH ARE NOT LISTED ABOVE

If you answered YES to any of the statements above, you probably lost too much blood in this cycle. It is recommended you see your doctor for check ups.

Before you go, Record the number of Pads or Tampons used in this Cycle in the Table below:

Day of Menses	# of Standard Pads used	Or Number of Tampons used	# Improvised Pads used
	SOAKED (x)	NOT SOAKED (y)	
Day 1			
Day 2			

Day 3			
Day 4			
Day 5			
Day 6			
Day 7			
	Total:	Total :	

Which of the Following Complaints did you experience 7 to 10 days before your menses?

1) Breast PAIN — YES/ NO
2) Vomiting — YES/NO
3) NAUSEA — YES/NO
4) HEADACHE — YES/NO
5) DEPRESSION or Feeling Low — YES/NO
6) LOSS OF APPETITE — YES/NO
7) CONSTIPATION — YES/NO
8) BACKACHE — YES/NO
9) ANGER — YES/NO
10) IRRITABLE — YES/NO
11) AGITATION — YES/NO

12) LACK OF SELF CONTROL   YES/NO
13) DIFFICULTIES WITH CONCENTRATION   YES/NO
14) TIREDNESS   YES/NO
15) INSOMNIA   YES/NO
16) I FEEL LUMPS IN MY BREASTS   YES/NO
17) WRITE OTHER COMPLAINTS YOU MAY EXPERIENCE WHICH ARE NOT LISTED ABOVE

If you answered YES to most of these statements, you probably experienced pre Menstrual tension or could be suffering from pre menstrual syndrome. Consult your gyneacologist for advice. See a Surgeon or Nurse for advice on Lumps in Your Breast.

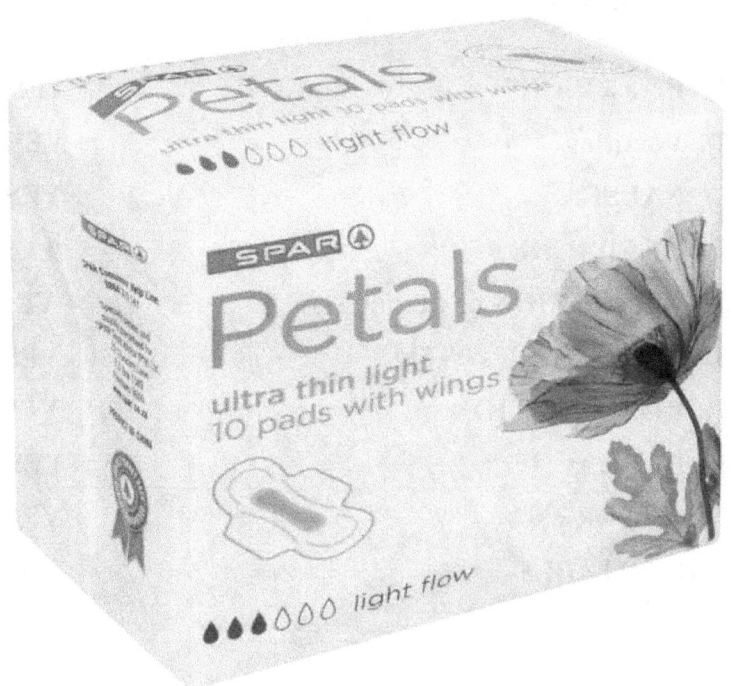

December 20......

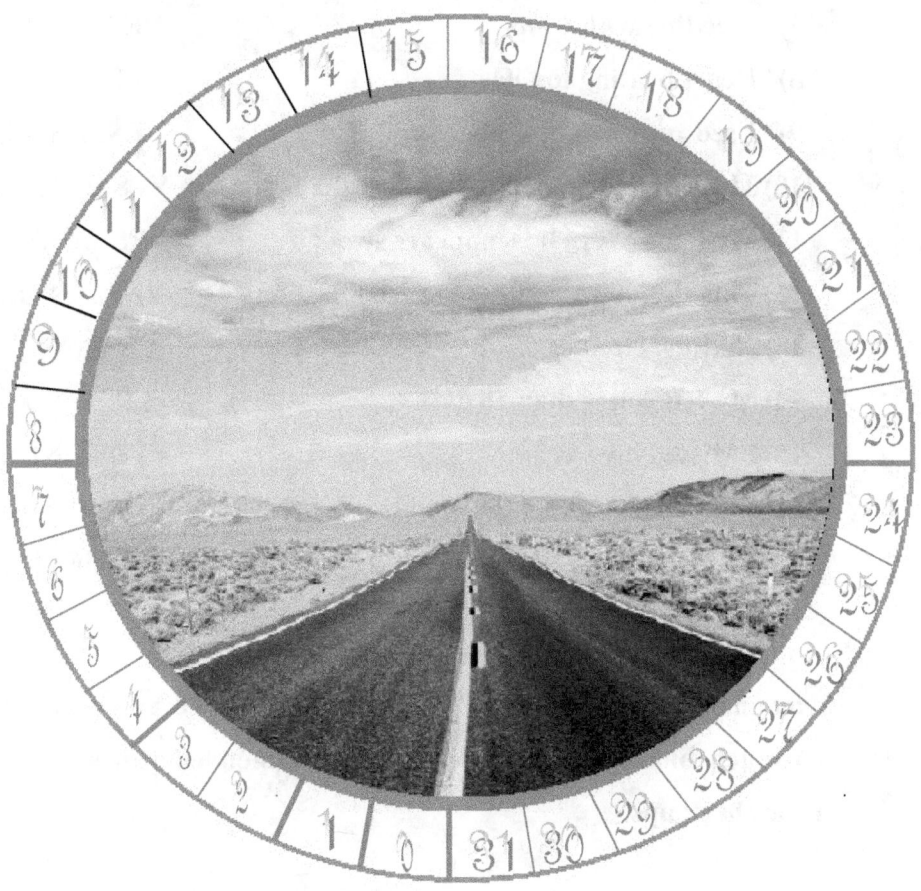

wHeEL

In this Cycle (Tick were appropriate)

1) Period lasted longer than seven days   YES... NO...
2) Used more pads than is usual for me   YES... NO...
3) Used more tampons than is usual for me   YES... NO...
4) I had very painful menses   YES... NO...

5) More pads soaked than is usual for me   YES... NO...
6) More tampons soaked than is usual for me   YES... NO...
7) Bleeding with Clots   YES... NO...
8) Heart beating too Fast   YES... NO...
9) Used Improvised Pads   YES... NO...
10) Menses made me ill & I missed the Exams   YES... NO ...
11) My Face & eye lids appears swollen   YES... NO...
12) This Period came too soon from last one   YES.... NO...
13) Getting Tired easily   YES...NO...
14) My HB is less than 10 g/dl   YES...NO...
15) I Missed my Period   YES...NO...
16) WRITE OTHER COMPLAINTS YOU MAY EXPERIENCE WHICH ARE NOT LISTED ABOVE

If you answered YES to any of the statements above, you probably lost too much blood in this cycle. It is recommended you see your doctor for check ups.

Before you go, Record the number of Pads or Tampons used in this Cycle in the Table below:

Day of Menses	# of Standard Pads used	Or Number of Tampons used	# Improvised Pads used
	SOAKED (x)	NOT SOAKED (y)	
Day 1			
Day 2			

Day 3			
Day 4			
Day 5			
Day 6			
Day 7			
	Total:	Total :	

Which of the Following Complaints did you experience 7 to 10 days before your menses?

1) Breast PAIN — YES/ NO
2) Vomiting — YES/NO
3) NAUSEA — YES/NO
4) HEADACHE — YES/NO
5) DEPRESSION or Feeling Low — YES/NO
6) LOSS OF APPETITE — YES/NO
7) CONSTIPATION — YES/NO
8) BACKACHE — YES/NO
9) ANGER — YES/NO
10) IRRITABLE — YES/NO
11) AGITATION — YES/NO

12) LACK OF SELF CONTROL YES/NO
13) DIFFICULTIES WITH CONCENTRATION YES/NO
14) TIREDNESS YES/NO
15) INSOMNIA YES/NO
16) I FEEL LUMPS IN MY BREASTS YES/NO
17) WRITE OTHER COMPLAINTS YOU MAY EXPERIENCE WHICH ARE NOT LISTED ABOVE

If you answered yes to most of these statements, you probably experienced pre Menstrual tension or could be suffering from pre menstrual syndrome. Consult your gyneacologist for advice. See a Surgeon or Nurse for advice on Lumps in Your Breast.

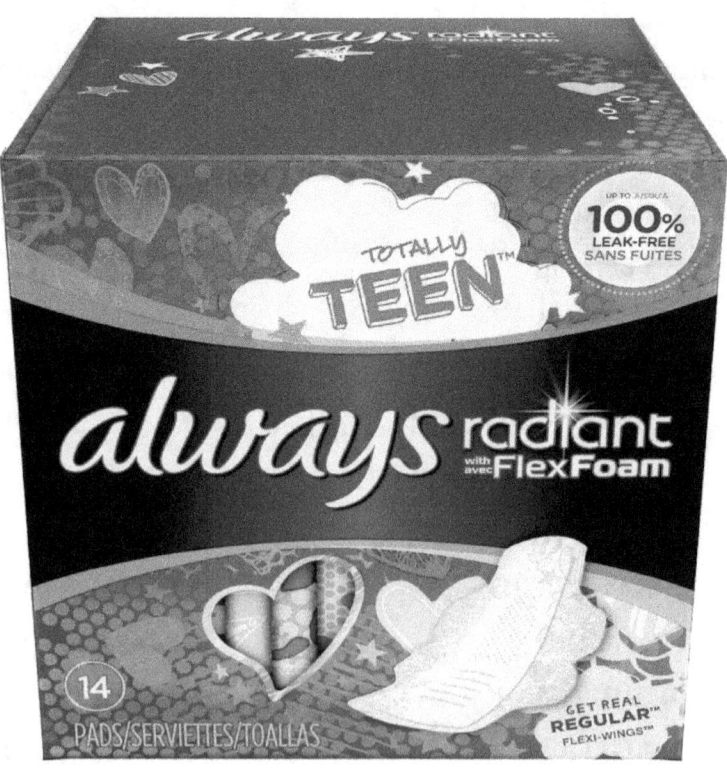

DID YOU KNOW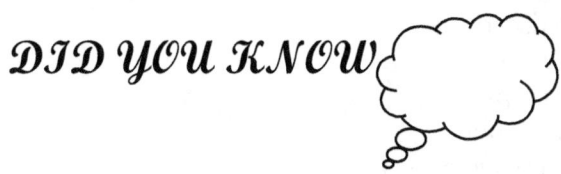

Metrorrhagia, also known as abnormal bleeding, is defined as bleeding in women that occurs between menstrual periods not associated with menstruation. This result in light to heavy bleeding that may or may not be accompanied by menstrual cramps.

Metrorrhagia is Uterine bleeding at irregular intervals, particularly between the expected menstrual periods. Metrorrhagia may be a sign of an underlying disorder, such as hormone imbalance, endometriosis, uterine fibroids or, less commonly, cancer of the uterus. Metrorrhagia may cause significant anemia. See also: Menometrorrhagia; Menorrhagia.

CAUSES OF ABNORMAL BLEEDING

There are various causes of abnormal bleeding. They may include the following:

- Hormonal imbalance
- Abnormal growths

- Pregnancy
- Miscarriage
- Fibroids
- Polyps
- Infection
- Cervical cancer
- Uterine cancer
- Types of birth control

Certain chronic medical conditions, such as thyroid disorders and diabetes can also cause abnormal bleeding. **(Continued on Page 95)**

SHOULD I WORRY ABOUT BREAST LUMPS

Though all breast lumps need to be evaluated by a trained medical professional, the majority turn out to be noncancerous, especially in younger women.

You're in the shower, conducting your monthly breast self-exam. Suddenly your hand freezes. You've found a lump. Now what?

First, don't panic, 80 to 85 percent of breast lumps are benign, meaning they are noncancerous, especially in women younger than age 40. Not only that, but if you're at an age where you've been having regular checkups, and if those checkups have been negative, you needn't worry about your palpable lump. It is not likely to be cancer.

But how do you know? How do you differentiate between a lump that is breast cancer and one that is Not; the so called benign lump? What causes benign breast lumps? And do they go away on their own?

Breast Lumps: Tell-Tale Distinctions

Your breasts are made up of fat, nerves, blood vessels, fibrous connective tissue, and glandular tissue, as well as an intricate milk-producing system of lobules (where the milk is made) and ducts (the thin tubes that carry milk to the nipple). This anatomy in and of itself creates a lumpy, uneven terrain.

A breast lump, however, distinguishes itself from this background of "normal" irregularities: A breast lump can be solid and unmovable like a dried bean, or soft and fluid-filled, rolling between your fingers like a grape. It can be smaller than a pea or BIGGER.

Meanwhile, what typically differentiates a benign breast lump from a cancerous breast lump is movement. A fluid-filled lump that rolls between the fingers is less likely to be cancer than a lump that is hard and rooted to the breast.

This is not to say all benign lumps move and all cancerous lumps don't. While this is a good rule of thumb, the only way to know for sure is through the wisdom of your doctor and specialized medical tests, such as an ultrasound, a mammogram, or a fine needle aspiration, in which your doctor uses a tiny needle to extract a bit of the lump for a biopsy, or laboratory examination. Another rule of thumb has to do with pain. Breast cancer does not usually present with pain, but benign conditions often do, although there are exceptions to this as well.

Not all benign breast lumps will require additional testing, by the way. If you find what appears to be a fluid-filled cyst during your menstrual period, your doctor may want to check your breast again at the end of your period to see if the cyst has disappeared. If the cyst goes away, you and your doctor will know your lump was indeed benign and related to the hormonal fluctuations associated with menstruation.

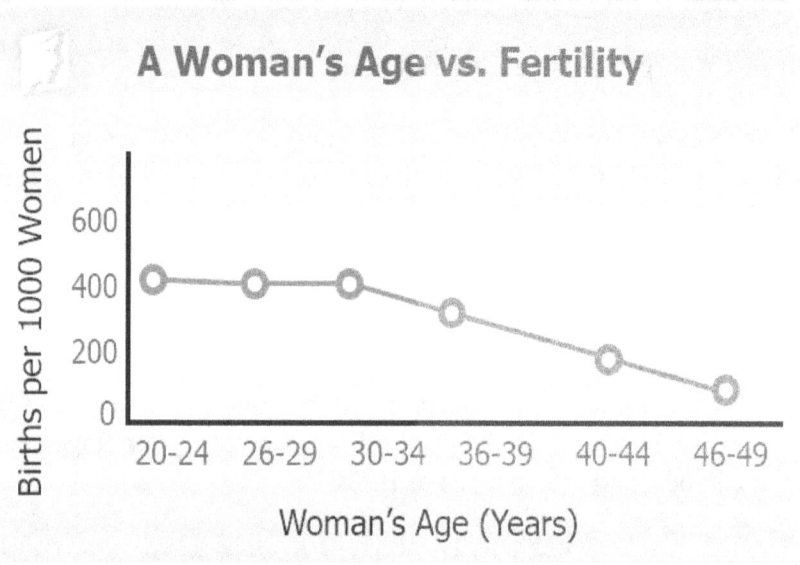

A Variety of Benign Breast Lumps and Conditions

Most benign breast lumps and conditions are directly related to your menstrual cycle — to fluctuations in your hormones and to the fluid build-up that comes with your monthly period. Other benign breast lumps and conditions may be related to plugged milk ducts, infections, and even breast injuries. Here are some of the most common benign breast conditions:

- **Fibroadenoma.** Occur in young girls and women in their teens and 20s. This benign tumor ranges in size from microscopic to several centimeters across. It is movable under the skin, round and hard like a marble, and may be diagnosed by aspiration or removal of the lump. If the Fibroadenoma shrinks or doesn't grow over time, and your doctor is sure of the diagnosis, he or she may decide to simply leave it alone.
- **Fibrocystic changes.** A general lumpiness that can be described as "ropy" or "granular," these lumps are the most commonly seen benign breast condition, affecting at least half of all women. Symptoms of fibrocystic change include pain, fibrous, rubbery tissue; a thickening of tissue; or a round, fluid-filled cyst. These changes, related to hormone fluctuation, may increase as you approach middle age and then disappear with menopause. Sometimes, your doctor will recommend limiting salt and caffeine in your diet to ease fluid build-up. You may also be prescribed hormones, in the form of birth control pills, to help ease particularly troublesome symptoms. Your doctor may also recommend a needle or surgical biopsy to make sure your breast condition is related to fibrocystic change and not cancer.
- **Cysts.** Related to fibrocystic changes, these are round or oval sacs, measuring one to centimeters across. They are painful to the touch and filled with fluid. They may come and go with your menstrual period, becoming larger and more painful at the beginning of your period and disappearing at the end. Your doctor may order an ultrasound or a fine needle aspiration to make sure it's a cyst and not something else. In very rare cases, when a cyst is particularly large or painful, your doctor may use a needle to withdraw and reduce the fluid inside it. Cysts generally affect women between the ages of 35 and 50.
- **Fat necrosis.** This occurs when fatty breast tissue is damaged by injury to the breast, resulting in the formation of round, firm lumps. It is more

common in women with large breasts, particularly in women who are obese. Your doctor will most likely watch the lump through several menstrual cycles and may decide to remove it surgically. Sometimes the necrosis will produce what is called an oily cyst, which your doctor will drain with a needle.
- **Nipple discharge.** Sometimes women experience nipple discharge with or without a breast lump. The color of nipple discharge related to benign fibrocystic changes can vary from yellow to green. A clear to milky discharge may mean a hormonal malfunction. Green-black discharge could be related to duct ectasia, a narrowing or blockage of the duct. It can even be bloody in appearance, which can, in fact, mean cancer. More than likely though, a red discharge means injury, infection, or a benign tumor. Your doctor may study the fluid under a microscope to determine its origin, particularly if there is also a mass or lump in your breast.
- **Mastitis.** An infection of the milk duct, this can create a lumpy, red, and warm breast, accompanied by fever. It occurs most commonly in women who are breastfeeding, but can occur in non-breastfeeding women as well. Treatment involves warm compresses and antibiotics.
- **Other less commonly known conditions.** Some medical conditions can also cause breast lumps, including hyperplasia, an overgrowth of cells in the breast ducts or lobules; adenosis, which causes enlarged lobules; intraductal papilloma, a wart-like growth of gland tissue that grows in the duct; and Lipoma which is a benign fatty tumor.

The risk for benign breast conditions increases for women who have never had children and those who have a history of irregular menstrual cycles and/or a family history of breast cancer.

If You Find a Breast Lump

All breast lumps should be evaluated by a medical professional, who will help you decide how to proceed. Most benign breast conditions are treatable, and some will even go away on their own, but it's best to let your doctor be the one to tell you that.

FIVE STEPS OF A BREAST SELF-EXAM

Step 1: Begin by looking at your breasts in the mirror with your shoulders straight and your arms on your hips.

Here's what you should look for:

- Breasts that are their usual size, shape, and color
- Breasts that are evenly shaped without visible distortion or swelling

If you see any of the following changes, bring them to your doctor's attention:

- Dimpling, puckering, or bulging of the skin
- A nipple that has changed position or an inverted nipple (pushed inward instead of sticking out)
- Redness, soreness, rash, or swelling

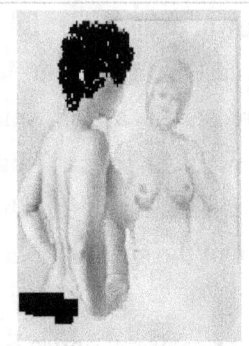

Breast Self-Exam — Step 1

Step 2: Now, raise your arms and look for the same changes.

Step 3: While you're at the mirror, look for any signs of fluid coming out of one or both nipples (this could be a watery, milky, or yellow fluid or blood).

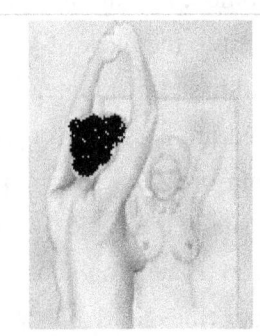

Step 4: Next, feel your breasts while lying down, using your right hand to feel your left breast and then your left hand to feel your right breast. Use a firm, smooth touch with the first few finger pads of your hand, keeping the fingers flat and together. Use a circular motion, about the size of a quarter.

Cover the entire breast from top to bottom, side to side — from your collarbone to the top of your abdomen, and from your armpit to your cleavage.

Follow a pattern to be sure that you cover the whole breast. You can begin at the nipple, moving in larger and larger circles until you reach the outer edge of the breast. You can also move your fingers up and down vertically, in rows, as if you were mowing a lawn. This up-and-down approach seems to work best for most women. Be sure to feel all the tissue from the front to the back of your breasts: for the skin and tissue just beneath, use light pressure; use medium pressure for tissue in the middle of your breasts; use firm pressure for the deep tissue in the back. When you've reached the deep tissue, you should be able to feel down to your ribcage.

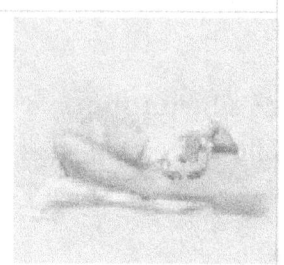

Breast Self-Exam — Step 4

Step 5: Finally, feel your breasts while you are standing or sitting. Many women find that the easiest way to feel their breasts is when their skin is wet and slippery, so they like to do this step in the shower. Cover your entire breast, using the same hand movements described in step 4.

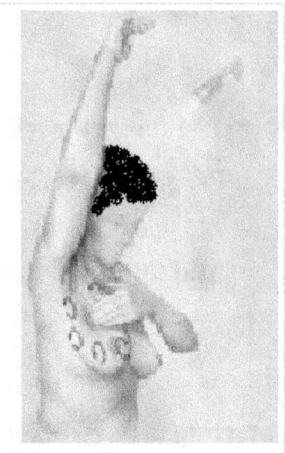

Breast Self-Exam — Step 5

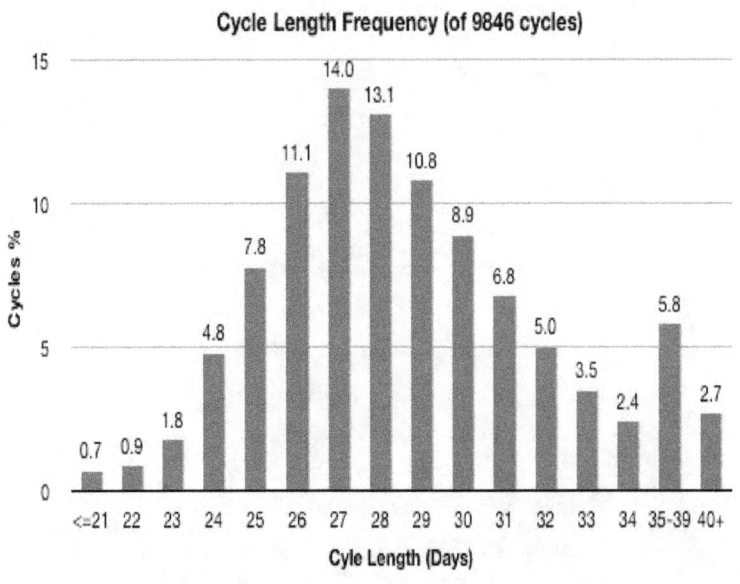

The danger period is the time in your cycle when you are likely to get Pregnant. It is estimated as follows;

Add 10 to the Last Day of your menses. This will give you the Day of your probable Ovulation. Sperms can survive for up to 72 hours inside a woman's body; the danger period therefore is the zone starting 3 days before the probable day of Ovulation and extending 3 days after the day of probable Ovulation.

However, there is no such a thing as SAFE DAYS. Every day is a Danger day when you have unsafe sex. You can contract many infections that are transmitted sexually even when you do not fall pregnant. These include; the Human Papilloma Virus which is associated with cervical cancer, the HIV virus, Zika Virus, Chlamydia infection, Gonorrhea, Syphilis, etc.

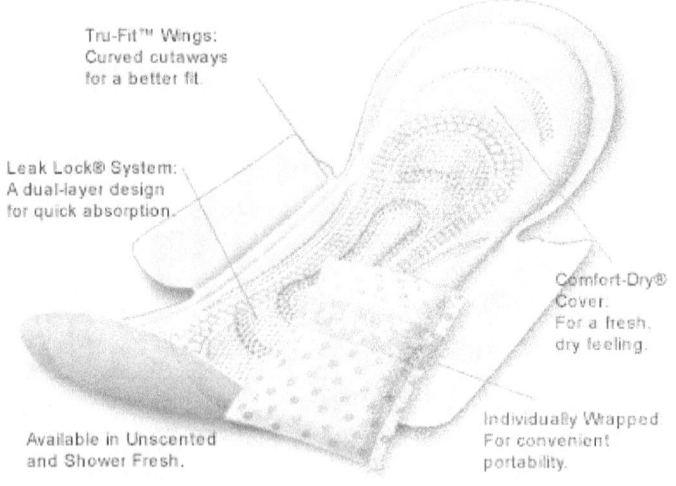

WARNING

USE OF NON STERILE IMPROVISED PADS IS UNHYGIENIC AND DANGEROUS. A Girl Child or Young Woman should <u>ONLY</u> Use Recommended/Standard Sterile Sanitary Pads or Tampons. A woman is at Greatest Risk to Ascending Pelvic infection during her Menses. This can lead to Pelvic Inflammatory Disease (PID) and may complicate into a Pelvic Abscess, Ectopic Pregnancy, chronic pelvic pain syndrome, Infertility later in life, etc. (Infertility is failure to conceive after a year of regular unprotected coitus usually referring to a married couple).

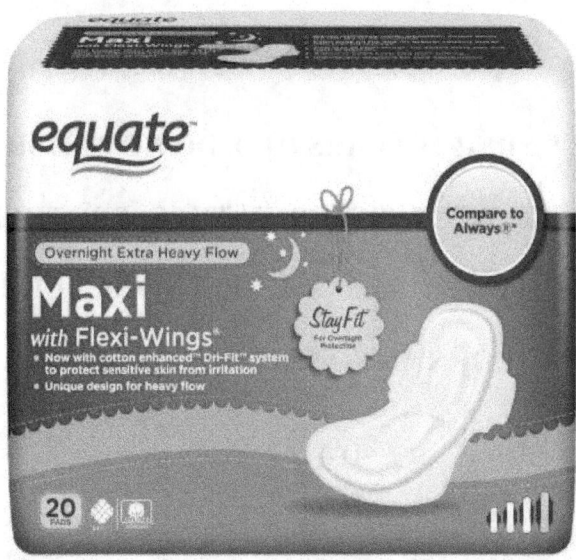

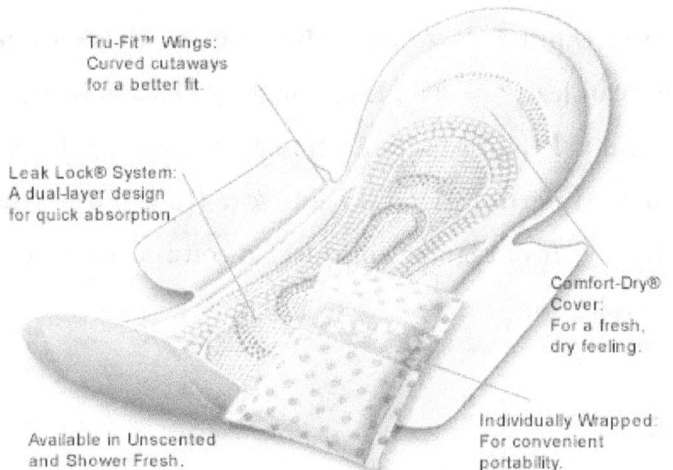

SHOW THIS BOOK TO YOUR HEALTH CARE PROVIDER DURING MENSTRUAL HEALTH CONSULTATION

***

IF YOU ARE UNDER 21 YEARS OLD, DO NOT BE SHY TO TELL YOUR MOTHER, AUNT, SISTER, FATHER, BROTHER, UNCLE, COUSIN and GRAND PARENTS ABOUT YOUR BUDGET FOR SANITARY PADS OR TAMPONS.

My First Experience, Where it found me

My name is Kay. This is my menstrual story when I was a little girl.

Growing up was great fun for me. We played lots of games as little girls. A deluge of memories flood my mind as I remember; Hide & Seek, Touch, Widaa, Start, Chidunu, Kamushi Kalilalila, Paada, Chiyenga, etc.

At eleven, I began to hear stories about girls bleeding when they grew up. I was scared at the stories older girls told us. Once, my friend Liz told her mother, one morning, that she was having dysentery each time she went to the bathroom. It turned out she was having menses. My friend certainly didn't know the difference between dysentery and Menses. She was only twelve at the time and her menses had just started. Like many young girls, menarche caught her unprepared.

There was, constantly, a level of secrecy surrounding the menstrual cycle. It was always very sad to see some of our friends mess up in class while the boys laughed and bullied these girls. Most teachers, unfortunately, were not very helpful to us the young girls. Some girls even went on to change schools because they couldn't stand being teased about the one time their uniforms were stained in class. The lessons about puberty come too late for many Girls. Our parents, in many families waited until the blood came.

The scanty knowledge I had about menses was from older girls that had already reached menarche. I also learnt a few things from my sister. Sometimes, we were fortunate to have talks in our school offered by personnel from a company that promoted use of sanitary pads. I always looked forward to the next visit by staff from this company. After each educational talk, they gave us sanitary pads. As useful as these talks were, unfortunately, they only allowed girls that had attained menarche to attend. I had not started my menses yet, however I always accompanied my friends who had started menses. I lied to the officials that I had attained menarche too just to be allowed into the school hall and learn. I gave the sanitary pads I was given to my sister.

I was fortunate the day my menses came; they found me on holiday from school. I woke up the morning of my 14th birthday and prepare for the day ahead. I felt a bit wet and thought I had wet the bed. I lifted my beddings and was horrified to see my white bed sheets soiled in blood. I was momentarily paralyzed by the shock that gripped my whole body. A torrent of tears rolled from my eyes. I didn't know what to do or whom to tell. My sister, Julian, was away on holiday. My mother was out of the country for school. There was only my uncle Joe at home that morning and my brother Phil.

I rushed to the bath room to check on my under wear. It was stained in blood. I sat on the toilet seat to pass urine and saw the water turn bloody. I couldn't tell whether I was passing bloody stained urine or having my menses. I thought I had bilharzia. I had heard people afflicted by this disease urinated blood. I was still in denial and cried quietly alone in the bathroom for some time. I do not remember how long I spent in the bath room that day. However, it was long enough to finish an entire roll of toilet paper.

After a while, I found I was not afraid any more. I had been told to share what was happening to me at that hour only with my aunt. Since she was not home and would not be home for a long time, I decided to keep quiet and not tell anyone what was happening to me. I was glad menarche had found me at home. I was delighted it did not find me in a class full of boys or on a bus. I was sad at the thought that many of the girls were not so fortunate. I dried my tears as my heart went out to all girls my age.

I decided to take a bath and clean myself. Then I sneaked into my mother's bedroom to look for her sanitary pads. I had always known where she hid her sanitary pads although she never talked to me about menses.

For the next week or so, I took care of myself and made sure no one found out I was having menses. My Aunt lived in another town and would be several months before she would come by to visit us.

The next time I bled, my elder sister found out and she confronted me. My secret was discovered and I was grounded. I was banned from handling food. I was banned from adding salt to food during the entire period of my menses. I was not allowed to go out and play with my friends, particularly with boys. I was told I could get pregnant if I played with bigger boys now that I had started menstruating. I was also told that if I cooked any food, those that would eat what I had cooked could fall ill. I was also told that adding salt to food could make everyone that ate the food suffer from Tuberculosis. I did not see the connection in all this.

However I could not question these traditional beliefs. I realized I had much to learn ahead.

When I grew up and got married and had my own daughter, I wanted things to be different for her. I would introduce issues shrouded in mystery about Menarche early in her life.

When the time came for her menses, it made things much easier for both of us. It was June 13th, 2006; she called me from the bathroom. I rushed to see what she was calling me for.

"Mom come and see," she called.

"I am here honey, what is the matter?" I asked when I got to the bathroom.

"Look," she said pointing to her soiled under pant on the floor.

She was not afraid. She stood there and smiled at me. I went over to her and put my arms around her. We sat in the bathroom and discussed what I had been telling her ever since she was seven.

"This may last a day or take up to seven days," I begun to explain.

"And I may experience abdominal pain and back ache. I may also experience headache and dizziness," she added.

"Headache and dizziness may be a sign that you have lost too much blood or that your blood was already low when the menses came," I explained.

"When this happens I will need to check my HB. My Hb should always be in the normal range. The normal range for girls and women is 11.5 to 16.5 grams per deciliter," she replied.

"That's correct," I answered.

"I will need to have pain killers incase the pain is severe. I will also need to have recommended sanitary pads at all times," she repeated what I had told her.

"I have sanitary pads in my wardrobe. I will show you how to wear a pad today," I explained with a smile.

"Am I allowed to cook and add salt to your food? Can I continue playing with John, the new boy in our class?" she asked and laughed.

We left the bathroom laughing. In my mind, I knew my daughter would never be the same again. She had a lot she still needed to learn ahead. The steps I took to teach her have since paid off. She has been able to help her cousins and friends at school.

***

Questions 1 - 22

Answer True (T) or False (F)

The following statements, Myths & Beliefs, concerning Menses, reproductive health & GBV are False

1. A girl on her menses should not be allowed to cook
2. A girl on her menses should not mix with people
3. When a Girl Child starts her menses, she ceases to be a girl. She becomes a woman.
4. When a Girl Child attains menarche, she transforms into a mature woman and can be married off by her parents.
5. A girl on her menses should not add salt to food to be eaten by others
6. A girl on her menses is unclean
7. When a girl on her menses adds salt to food, those that eat the food will develop a cough that has no cure
8. A girl that has started having menses can fall pregnant when she has sex with a boy or man
9. A girl on her menses should stay in her bedroom till menses end
10. A girl on her menses should not go to school till her periods end
11. A girl on her menses should eat alone and should be saved food by only one person.
12. Some girls start menses as early as nine years of age
13. A new born Girl Baby can have menses
14. Girls mature earlier than boys
15. Menses do not cause mood swings in the life of Girls and Women
16. The Moon is not responsible for mood swings seen during menses
17. A Girl should undergo sexual cleansing when she starts her first menses to prevent diseases and misfortunes in the family

18. A man who touches a Girl Child's Breasts, Legs or Buttocks in a sexual manner commits Indecent Assault and should be imprisoned upon conviction for a term of NOT less than Fourteen years.
19. A 16year old Boy who commits Indecent Assault on a 16 year old Girl is liable to 20 years imprisonment upon conviction.
20. Any person who conducts or causes to be conducted a harmful cultural practice on a child commits a felony and is liable, upon conviction, to imprisonment to a term not less than fifteen years and maybe liable to imprisonment for life.
21. Indecent Assault is a crime of touching another person in a sexual manner without consent, or where the person lacks capacity to give consent.
22. An Uncle or Teacher fondling or kissing a 15yr old Girl is not guilty of Indecent Assault if the Girl agreed to be touched in a sexual manner

Answer sheet Q2030

Tick where appropriate

1. T...F...	13) T...F...
2. T...F...	14) T...F...
3. T...F...	15) T...F...
4. T...F...	16) T...F...
5. T...F...	17) T...F...
6. T...F...	18) T...F...
7. T...F...	19) T...F...
8. T...F...	20) T...F...
9. T...F...	21) T...F...
10. T...F...	22) T...F...
11. T...F...	23) T...F...
12. T...F...	24) T...F...

GBV and You
Gender Based Violence (GBV)

Here is what every Girl, Lady and young Woman should know;

Anti- Gender Based Violence Act of 2010 is an ACT of Parliament of Zambia which was passed to protect victims and survivors of Gender- based violence;

It is written in Chapter 87 of the Laws used for dealing with Crime and Punishment in Zambia;

A Sexual Offender is Liable, upon conviction of Defilement or Rape, to imprisonment for a term not less than Fifteen years and maybe liable to imprisonment for LIFE.

You will be delighted to learn the various punishments Law breakers of sexual offenses will dance to when you report them. Here are some interesting sections of the Law for your reference.

SECTION 131

Definition of Child

In this part "Child" means a person below the age of sixteen (16) years.

SECTION 132

RAPE

Any person who, has unlawful carnal knowledge of a woman or girl, without her consent or with the consent; If the consent is obtained by force or means of threats or intimidation of any kind by force or fear of bodily harm or by means of false representation as to the nature of the act or in case of married woman, by personating her husband, is guilty of a felony termed rape and is liable to imprisonment for life.

Attempted Rape Contrary to section 134:

Anyone who attempts to commit rape is guilty of a felony and liable to imprisonment for life.

SECTION 137

Indecent Assault

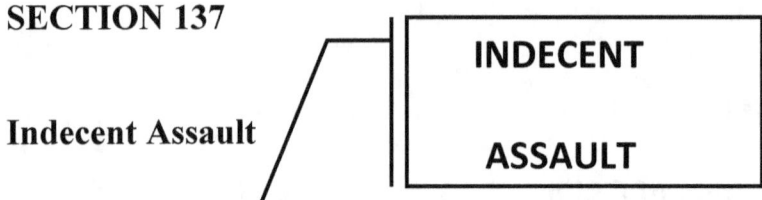

1. Any person who unlawfully and indecently assaults any child or other person commits a felony and is liable, upon conviction, to imprisonment for a term of not less than fourteen years and not exceeding twenty years.
2. **It shall NOT be a defense to a charge of an indecent assault on a child to prove that the child consented to the act of indecency.**
3. Any person who is found in a building or dwelling house or in any veranda or passage attached thereto or in any yard, garden or other land adjacent to or within the cartilage of such building or dwelling house not being a public place:
    a. For the purpose of and from motives of indecent curiosity gazing at or observing any other person or child who may be therein while in a state of undress or semi-undress; or
    b. With intent to annoy or indecently to assault any child or other person who may be there;

Commits an Offence and is liable, upon conviction, to imprisonment

for a term of not less than two years and not exceeding five years.

SECTION 137A

Sexual Harassment

SEXUAL HARASSMENT

4. Any person who practices sexual harassment in a work place, institution of learning or elsewhere on a child commits a felony and is liable, upon conviction, to imprisonment to a term of not less than three years and not exceeding fifteen years.
5. A Child who commits an offence under section (1) is liable to such community service or counseling as the court may determine in the best interest of the child.
6. In this section, sexual harassment means;

   e. A seductive sexual advance being unsolicited sexual comment, physical contact or other gesture of a sexual nature which one finds objectionable or offensive or causes discomfort in one's studies or job and interferes with academic performance or work performance or a conducive working environment or study environment;
   f. Sexual bribery in the form of soliciting or attempting to solicit sexual activity by promise of reward;
   g. Sexual threat or coercion which includes procuring or attempting to procure sexual activity by threat of violence or victimization or;
   h. Sexual imposition using forceful behavior or assault in an attempt to gain physical sexual contact.

SECTION 138

DEFILEMENT OF A CHILD

1. Any person who unlawfully and carnally knows any child commits a felony and is liable upon conviction, to a term of imprisonment of not less than fifteen (15) years and maybe be liable to imprisonment for life.
2. Any person who attempts to have unlawful carnal knowledge of any child commits a felony and is liable, upon conviction, to imprisonment for a term not less than fourteen (14) years and not exceeding twenty years.
3. Any person who prescribes a defilement of a child as cure for any ailment commits a felony and is liable, upon conviction to imprisonment of not less than fifteen (15) years and maybe liable to imprisonment for life.
4. A Child above the age of twelve who commits an offence under sub-section (1) or (2) is liable, to such community service or counseling as the court may determine, in the best interest of both children.

SECTION 139

Defilement of an imbecile or person with mental illness

Any person who, knowing a child or other person to be an imbecile or a person with mental illness, has or attempts to have unlawful carnal knowledge of that child or other person in circumstances not amounting to rape, but which prove that the offender knew at the time of the commission of the offence that the child or the other person was an idiot or imbecile commits a felony and is liable, upon conviction, to imprisonment for a term not less than fourteen (14) years.

SECTION 140

Procuring a Child or Other Person for Prostitution, etc

Any person who;

Procures or attempts to procure any child or other person to have unlawful carnal knowledge either in Zambia or elsewhere, with any person or other persons for pornography, bestiality or any other purposes;

a. Procures or attempts to procure any child or other person to become, either in Zambia or elsewhere, a common prostitute;
b. Procures or attempts to procure any child or person to leave Zambia, with the intent that the child or person may become an inmate or frequent a brothel elsewhere or;
c. Procures or attempts to procure any child or person to leave that child's other person's usual place of abode in Zambia with intent that the child or other person may, for the purpose of prostitution, become an inmate of or frequent a brothel either in Zambia or elsewhere;

Commits a felony and is liable, upon conviction, to imprisonment for a term of not less than twenty years and may be liable to imprisonment for life;

Provided that no person shall be convicted of an offence under this section upon the evidence or one witness only, unless such witness be corroborated in some material particular by evidence implicating the accused.

SECTION 142

Householder, etc

Permitting Defilement of Child on Premises

Any person who, being the owner or occupier of premises or having or acting or assisting in the management or control thereof, induces or knowingly permits any child to resort to or be upon such premises for the purpose of being unlawfully and carnally known by any other person, commits a felony and is liable, upon conviction, to imprisonment for not less than twenty (20) years and maybe liable to imprisonment for life.

SECTION 143

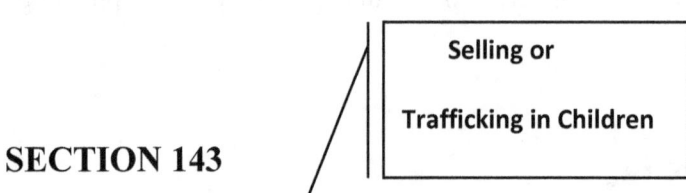

Selling or Trafficking in Children

Any person who sells or traffics in a child or other for any purpose or in any form commits an offence and is liable, upon conviction, to imprisonment for a term not less than twenty (20) years;

- ✓ Provided that where it is proved during the trial of the accused person that the sell or trafficking in a child or other person was for the purpose of causing that the child or person to be unlawfully and carnally known by any other person, whether such carnal knowledge was intended to be with any person or generally, the person is liable upon conviction, to imprisonment for life.
- ✓ However, in 2008 the law was enacted to specifically deal with human trafficking Act No. 11 of 2008

SECTION 144

Detention with Intent or in a Brothel

1. Any person who detains any child or other person against that child or other person's will;
    a. In or upon any premises with intent that the child or other person may be unlawfully and carnally known by any third person, whether particularly or generally or for rituals or any other purposes or
    b. In a brother

Commits a felony and is liable, upon conviction, to imprisonment for a term of not less than twenty (20) years and may be liable to imprisonment for life.

2. When a child or person is in or upon any premises for the purposes of having any unlawful carnal knowledge or is in any brothel, another person shall be deemed to detain such a child or persons in or upon such premises or in such brothel, if, with intent to compel or induce the child or person to remain in or upon such premises or in such brothel, such other person withholds from the child or person any wearing apparel or other property belonging to the child or person or where wearing apparel has been lent or otherwise supplied to such child or person or by the directions of such person, such other person threatens such person with legal proceedings for taking away the wearing apparel so lent or supplied.

3. No legal proceedings, whether civil or criminal, shall be taken against any child or person for taking away or being found in possession of any such wearing apparel as was necessary to enable the child or person to leave such premises or brothel.

SECTION 150

Conspiracy to defile

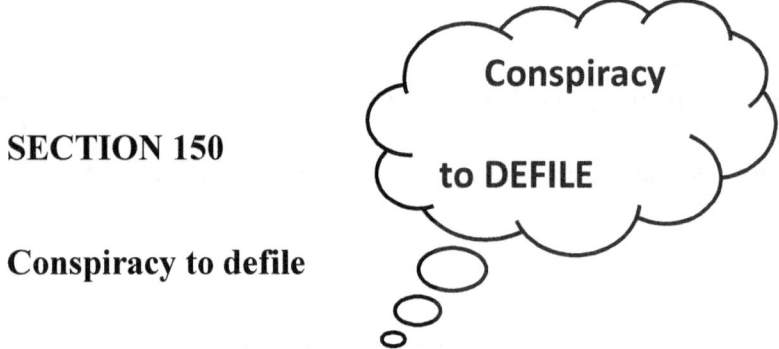

Any person who conspires with another person to induce any person or child, by means of any false pretence or other fraudulent means, to permit any other person to have unlawful carnal knowledge of such person or child, commits a felony and liable, upon conviction, to imprisonment for a term of not less than fifteen years and may be liable to imprisonment for life.

SECTION 155

Unnatural Offences

a. Has carnal knowledge of any person against the order of nature
b. Has carnal knowledge of an animal
c. Permit a male person to have carnal knowledge of him or her against the order of nature is guilty of a felony and liable to imprisonment for fourteen (14) years.

SECTION 156

Attempt to commit unnatural offences

Any person who attempts to commit any of these offences specified in section 155 commits a felony and is liable, upon conviction, to imprisonment for a term not less than fifteen seven years but not exceeding fourteen years.

SECTION 157

Harmful Cultural Practices

1. Any person who conducts or causes to be conducted a harmful cultural practice on a child commits a felony and is liable, upon conviction, to imprisonment to a term not less than fifteen years and maybe liable to imprisonment for life.
2. In this section (harmful cultural practice) includes sexual cleansing, female genital mutilation or an initiation ceremony that results in injury, the transmission of an infectious or life threatening disease or loss of life to a child but does not include circumcision on a male child.

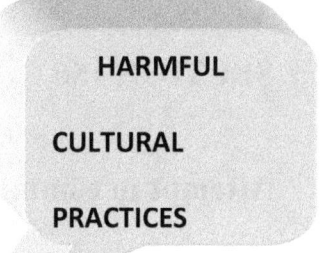

Here is an Example of Harmful Cultural Practices in Africa

In some remote southern regions of Malawi, it's a tradition for girls to be made to have sex with a paid sex worker known as a "Hyena" once they reach puberty. The act is not seen by village elders as rape, but as a form of ritual "cleansing".

I meet Eric Aniva in the dusty yard of his three-room shack in Nsanje district in southern Malawi. Goats and Chickens graze in the dirt outside. Wearing a grimy green shirt, and walking with a pronounced limp (he's been lame in one leg since birth, he says), he greets me enthusiastically. He seems to like the idea of media attention.

Aniva is by all accounts the pre-eminent "hyena" in this village. It is a traditional title given to a man hired by the communities in several remote parts of southern Malawi to provide what is called sexual "cleansing". If a man dies, for example, his wife is required by tradition to sleep with Aniva before she can bury him. If a woman has an abortion, again sexual cleansing is required.

And most shockingly, in Nsanje, teenage girls, after their first menstruation, are made to have sex over a three –day period, to mark their passage from childhood to womanhood. If the girls refuse, it is believed, disease or some fatal misfortune could befall their families or the village as a whole.

"Most of those I have slept with are girls, school going girls," Aniva tells me. "Some girls are just 12 or 13 years old, but I prefer them older. All these girls find pleasure in having me as their hyena. They actually are proud and tell other people that this man, is a real man, he knows how to please a woman."

Despite his boast, several girls I meet in a nearby village express aversion to the ordeal they've had to go through.

"There was nothing else I could have done. I had to do it for the sake of my parents," one girl, Maria, tells me. "If I'd refused, my family members could be attacked with diseases, even death, so I was scared."

They tell me that all their female friends were made to have sex with a hyena.

Aniva appears to be in his 40s (he's vague about his precise age) and currently has two wives who are well aware of his work. He claims to have slept with over 104 women and girls- although he said the same to a local newspaper in 2012, I sense that he long ago lost count. Aniva has five children that he knows about. He is not sure how many of the women and girls he's made pregnant.

He tells me, he is one of ten hyenas in this community, and that every village in Nsanje has them. The hyenas are paid $4 to $7 each time.

An hour's drive down the road, I'm introduced to Fagisi, Chrissie and Phelia, women in their 50s and custodians of the initiation traditions in their village. It's their job to organize the adolescent girls into camps each year, teaching them about their duties as wives and how to please a man sexually. The "sexual cleansing" with the hyena is the final stage of this process, arranged voluntarily by the girl's parents. "It's necessary," Fagisi, Chrissie and Phelia explain, "to avoid disease befalling their parents and the rest of the village."

"We have to train our girls in a good manner in the village, so that they don't go astray, are good wives so that the husband is satisfied," Chrissie tells me.

I put it to them that there's a much greater risk that these "cleansing" will themselves spread disease. According to custom, sex with the hyena must never be protected with the use of condoms. But they say a hyena is hand –picked for his good morals, and therefore cannot be infected with HIV/Aids.

It is clear, given the hyena's duties, that HIV is a huge risk to the community. The UN estimates that one in ten of all Malawians carry the virus. So I ask Aniva if he is HIV positive. He astounds me by saying that he is HIV positive and that he doesn't mention this to a girl's parents when they hire him.

(This man was arrested soon after this bizarre custom was revealed)

***

Defilement or Conspiracy to defile

Any person who conspires with another person to induce any person or child, by means of any false pretence or other fraudulent means, to permit any other person to have unlawful carnal knowledge of such person or child, commits a felony and liable, upon conviction, to imprisonment for a term of not less than fifteen years and may be liable to imprisonment for life.

The Law is clear in Zambia….. Report any such Hyenas to the Police

Some Words You should Know

- **Carnal Knowledge** – Sexual intercourse between a male and female in which there is at least some slight penetration of the woman's vagina by the man's penis
- **Felony** – A serious offense or crime. E.g. murder or rape
- **Misdemeanor**- Offenses lower than felonies and generally those punishable by fine, penalty or simple imprisonment.
- **Rape** - Any act of sexual intercourse that is forced upon a person
- **Defilement**- the act of having sexual intercourse with a child
- **Child**- A person aged below sixteen (16) years of age
- **Consent**- permission for something to happen or agreement to do something
- **Liable**- answerable or legally responsible for something.
- **Indecent assault**- sexual assault that does not involve rape. It is a crime of touching another person in a sexual manner without consent, or where the person lacks capacity to give consent. Indecent assault is an offense of aggravated assault.
- **Aggravated assault**- A person is guilty of aggravated assault if he or she attempts to cause serious bodily injury to another or causes such injury purposely, knowingly, or recklessly under circumstances manifesting extreme indifference to the value of human life.
- **Indecent assault**- Under the Zambian penal code Act, Chapter 87; any person who unlawfully and **indecently assaults** any woman or girl is guilty of a felony and is liable to imprisonment for **fourteen years**.
- **Bestiality**- sex between a person and an animal
- **Sexual Intercourse**- sexual contact between individuals involving penetration, especially the insertion of a man's erect penis into a woman's vagina (known as vaginal intercourse), typically culminating in orgasm and the ejaculation of semen; for pleasure, reproduction or both.
- **Bestiality**- sex between a person and an animal. E.g. a human having sex with a dog
- **Next of Friend** – is a person who represents another person who is under disability or otherwise unable to maintain a suit on his or her own behalf who does not have a legal guardian.

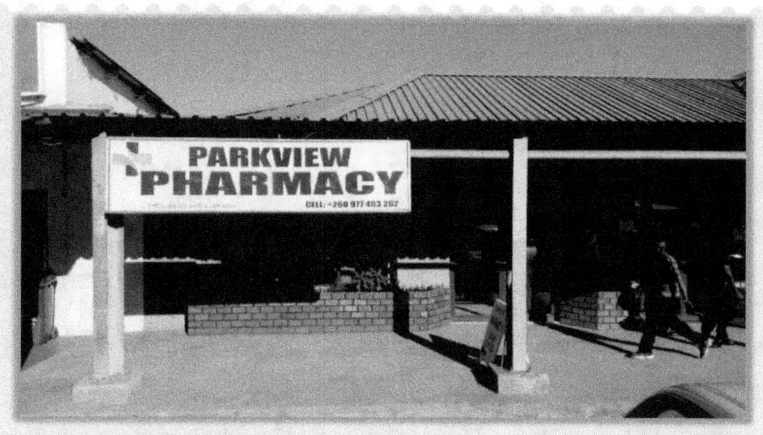

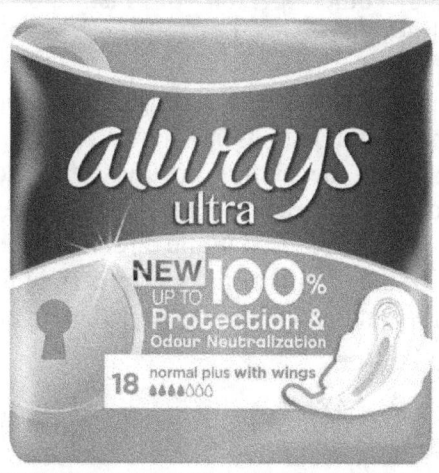

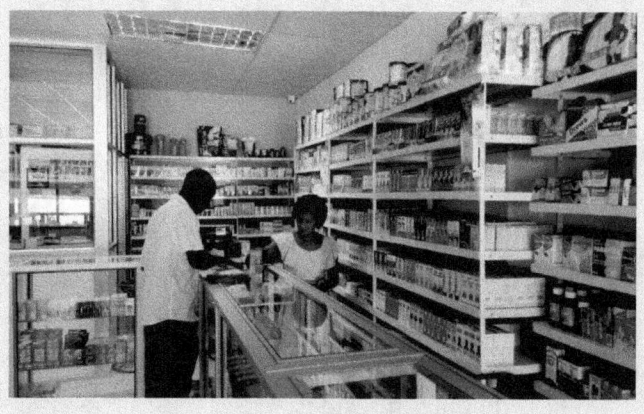

GBV INFORMATION FOR YOU

FILING OF, AND DEALING WITH, COMPLAINTS OF GENDER-BASED VIOLENCE

4. A single act may amount to gender-based violence.

5. A police officer, labour inspector, social worker, counselor, medical practitioner, legal practitioner, nurse, religious leader, traditional leader, teacher, employer or other person or institution with information concerning the commission of an act of gender-based violence shall;

    (a) Inform a victim of the victim's rights and any basic support which may be available to assist the victim;

    (b) Obtain for the victim, or advise the victim how to obtain shelter, medical treatment, legal services, counseling or other service that may be required in the circumstances; and

    (c) Advice the victim of the victim's right to lodge a complaint against the respondent including remedies available to the victim under this Act.

6.

(1) A victim of gender-based violence may file a complaint about the gender-based violence.

(2) A child or a person with a mental disability may be assisted by a next friend to file a complaint of gender-based violence.

(3) Notwithstanding subsection (1), a complaint of gender-based violence may be filed by any other person or institution with information about the gender-based violence where the intervention is in the interest of the victim.

(4) A complaint of gender-based violence shall be filed with the police at the place;

    (a) Where the offender resides;
    (b) Where the victim resides;

(c) Where the gender-based violence occurred or is occurring or is likely to occur;

(d) If the victim has left the victim's usual place of abode, where the victim is residing temporarily; or

(e) that is convenient for the person filing the complaint.

7. A police officer shall respond promptly to a request by any person for assistance from gender-based violence and shall offer such protection as the circumstances of the case or the person who made the report requires even when the person reporting is not the victim of the gender-based violence.

8. (1) where a police officer receives a complaint under subsection (4) of section six, the police officer shall;

(a) Interview the parties and witnesses to the gender-based violence;

(b) Record the complaint in detail and provide the victim with an extract of the complaint, upon request, in a language the victim understands;

(c) assist the victim to obtain medical treatment, where necessary;

(d) assist the victim to a place of safety as the circumstances of the case or as the victim requires where the victim expresses concern about safety;

(e) protect the victim to enable the victim retrieve personal belongings, where applicable; and

(f) assist and advise the victim to preserve evidence.

(2) Where one of the parties or witnesses to an act of gender-based violence, a complaint of which has been made under subsection (4) of section six, is a child, a police officer who receives the complaint shall interview the child in the presence of;

(a) the parent or guardian of the child; or

(b) a next friend, where the parent or guardian is the respondent.

(3) Police assistance to a victim under paragraph (c) of subsection (1) consists of issuing a medical form to the victim and, where necessary, sending the victim to a health facility.

(4) A victim of gender-based violence who is assisted by the police to obtain medical treatment under paragraph (c) of subsection (1), shall be entitled to free medical treatment at a public health facility and a free medical report within a reasonable period of time.

(5) Family mediation or intervention shall not be a bar to the investigation or prosecution of a complaint of gender-based violence.

(6) For the purposes of this section, "health facility" has the meaning assigned to it in the Health Professions Act, 2009.

9. A police officer may, without a warrant, arrest a person where the police officer has reasonable grounds to believe that the person;

(a) is committing, or has committed, an offence under this Act;
(b) is about to commit an offence under this Act and there is no other way to prevent the commission of the offence;
(c) unless arrested, will;
  (i) escape or cause an unreasonable delay, trouble or expense in being made answerable to justice;
  (ii) interfere with the witnesses; or
  (iii) tamper with, or destroy, relevant evidence or material;
(d) is willfully obstructing the police officer in the execution of police duties; or

(e) has contravened or is contravening an order issued under this Act.

DID YOU KNOW?

Metrorrhagia: Uterine bleeding at irregular intervals, particularly between the expected menstrual periods. Metrorrhagia may be a sign of an underlying disorder, such as hormone imbalance, endometriosis, uterine fibroids or, less commonly, cancer of the uterus. Metrorrhagia may cause significant anemia. See also: Menometrorrhagia; Menorrhagia.

CAUSES OF ABNORMAL BLEEDING

There are various causes of abnormal bleeding. They may include the following:

- Hormonal imbalance
- Abnormal growths
- Pregnancy
- Miscarriage

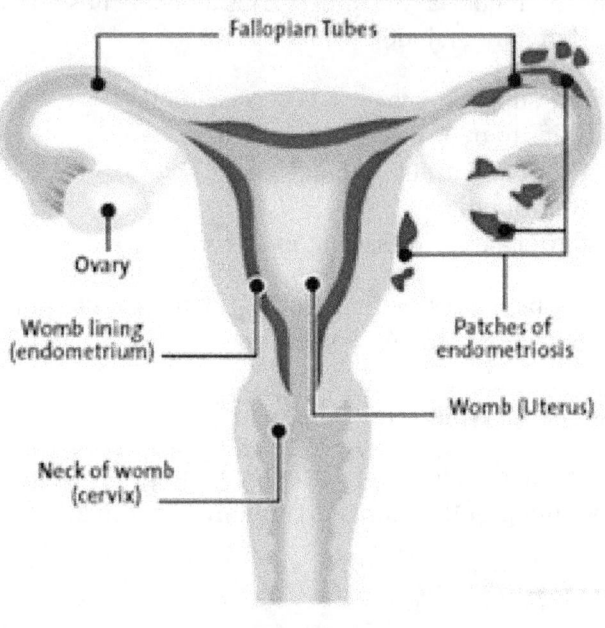

- Fibroids
- Polyps
- Infection
- Cervical cancer
- Uterine cancer
- Types of birth control

Certain chronic medical conditions, such as thyroid disorders and diabetes can also cause abnormal bleeding.

DIAGNOSIS OF ABNORMAL BLEEDING

To diagnose the cause of this condition, the doctor will evaluate the patient's medical history, including the frequency and length of menstrual periods. Additional tests to examine blood and the uterus may include:

- Blood tests
- Ultrasound
- Endometrial biopsy
- Hysteroscopy

TREATMENT OF ABNORMAL BLEEDING

Treatment for abnormal bleeding varies and depends on the cause of the condition, but may include:

- Hormone supplements
- Antibiotics to treat infection
- Removal of an intrauterine device
- Birth control pills
- Non-steroidal anti-inflammatory medication

Surgery may be necessary to remove growths such as polyps or fibroids that can cause bleeding. Other types of surgery may include:

- **Endometrial Ablation**

Endometrial ablation is a procedure that may be performed to destroy the lining of the uterus to minimize or stop bleeding.

- **Hysterectomy**

In severe cases, a hysterectomy may be recommended. This is a surgical procedure that removes the entire uterus. A hysterectomy requires a hospital stay and involves a long recovery.

Abnormal bleeding should be treated based on underlying causes and the patient's individual condition. Metrorrhagia caused by a miscarriage requires prompt medical attention to prevent serious complications.

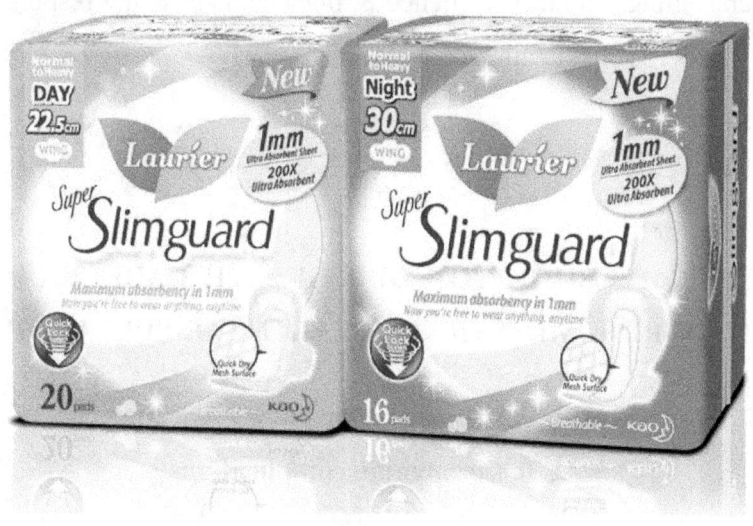

***

The Adolescent Girl Child needs special education to understand the hormonal storm raging inside her young and naive body. Everyone expects her to hurriedly learn to manage herself and navigate the complex world around her. She is often judged harshly when she stumbles and falls.

The menstrual cycle causes her to lose blood every Month. This may cause her Anemia, a medical condition that is characterized by; poor concentration, headaches, dizziness, weakness, getting tired easily, reduced mental capacity, low immunity, poor wound healing, poor appetite, lethargy, fainting, heart failure, poor oxygen delivery to body organs, poor skin health, poor performance in school, etc.

The Menstrual Cycle is Central to Women's Health in Everyday Life; its understanding, monthly vigilance & management, is the responsibility of every Lady, Woman and the Girl Child.

***

SHOW THIS BOOK TO YOUR HEALTH CARE PROVIDER DURING MENSTRUAL HEALTH CONSULTATION

Ask your Health Care Provider how Anemia can lead to Life threatening complications

www.ingramcontent.com/pod-product-compliance
Lightning Source LLC
Chambersburg PA
CBHW060358190526
45169CB00002B/648